Sperm Banking

Sperm Banking: Theory and Practice

Edited by

Allan A. Pacey
University of Sheffield

Mathew J. Tomlinson
Nottingham University Hospital

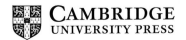

CAMBRIDGE UNIVERSITY PRESS
Cambridge, New York, Melbourne, Madrid, Cape Town, Singapore,
São Paulo, Delhi

Cambridge University Press
The Edinburgh Building, Cambridge CB2 8RU, UK

Published in the United States of America by
Cambridge University Press, New York

www.cambridge.org
Information on this title: www.cambridge.org/9780521611282

© Cambridge University Press 2009

First published 2009

Printed in the United Kingdom at the University Press, Cambridge

A catalogue record for this publication is available from the British Library

ISBN 978-0-521-61128-2 paperback

Contents

Contributors   vi
Preface   vii
Acknowledgements   viii

1. **The history of sperm cryopreservation**   1
   Eric M. Walters, James D. Benson, Erik J. Woods, and John K. Critser

2. **Effects of antineoplastic and other medical treatments on sperm production**   18
   Marvin L. Meistrich

3. **Referring patients for sperm banking**   30
   Allan A. Pacey

4. **The psychological and psychosocial issues surrounding sperm banking**   41
   Marilyn A. Crawshaw

5. **Legal and ethical aspects of sperm banking**   58
   Susan Avery

6. **Methods of sperm retrieval and banking in cancer patients**   73
   Sepideh Mehri, Jose Sepulveda, and Pasquale Patrizio

7. **Sperm processing and storage**   86
   Mathew J. Tomlinson

8. **Assisted reproduction using banked sperm**   105
   Hasan M. El-Fakahany and Denny Sakkas

9. **Future developments for fertility preservation in men**   115
   Mathew J. Tomlinson and Allan A. Pacey

Index   122

Contributors

Susan Avery
Assisted Conception Unit,
Birmingham Women's Hospital,
Birmingham, UK.

James D. Benson
Comparative Medicine Center,
College of Veterinary Medicine,
University of Missouri, Columbia,
USA.

Marylin A. Crawshaw
Department of Social Policy & Social
Work, University of York,
Heslington, UK.

John K. Critser
Comparative Medicine Center,
College of Veterinary Medicine,
University of Missouri, Columbia,
USA.

Hasan M. El-Fakahany
Dermatology, STDs, and Andrology
Department Al-Minya
University Hospital, Al-Minya, Egypt.

Sepideh Mehri
Yale University Fertility Centre
New Haven, USA.

Marvin L. Meistrich
Department of Experimental Radiation
Oncology, The University of Texas
M. D. Anderson Cancer Center,
Houston, USA.

Allan A. Pacey
Academic Unit of Reproductive and
Developmental Medicine,
University of Sheffield, UK.

Pasquale Patrizio
Yale University Fertility Centre,
New Haven, USA.

Denny Sakkas
Yale University School of Medicine,
New Haven, USA.

Jose Sepulveda
Istituto Etudio Concepcion Humana,
Monterrey, Mexico.

Mathew J. Tomlinson
Fertility Unit, Nottingham University
Hospital, Nottingham, UK.

Eric M. Walters
Comparative Medicine Center,
College of Veterinary Medicine,
University of Missouri, Columbia,
USA.

Erik J. Woods
Genome Resources, Indianapolis, USA.

Preface

Sperm banking is now routinely offered to men as a means of preserving their fertility prior to either medical or surgical treatments that have a high risk of rendering them infertile. This is most common before cancer treatments such as chemo- or radiotherapy but is becoming increasingly common in other areas of medicine that rely on the use of potentially cytotoxic drugs, including the treatments for autoimmune conditions or in cases of progressive loss of muscular or neurological function. Some men elect to bank sperm prior to surgery, either because the surgery is intended as a contraceptive measure (e.g. vasectomy) or because infertility is an unwanted side effect of the operation. Lastly, and less commonly, men are now wishing to preserve their fertility as a precautionary measure because of a high-risk occupation or activity, including service in the security or armed forces. Whilst this book deals primarily with sperm banking prior to planned medical treatments with gonadotoxic agents, the processes involved are largely similar whatever the reason for wanting to bank sperm.

Despite sperm banking now being routine in almost every major city throughout the world, very little has been written about the clinical process from beginning to end. Only technical details about the freezing of sperm, the effects of certain cytotoxic treatments on male fertility, or the number of men coming forward to use banked samples have been described in individual research papers. This was highlighted at a one-day workshop in May 2002, organized by the British Andrology Society in Birmingham, UK. At that meeting, a series of presentations and open forum discussions, the idea that sperm banking was a unique service in its own right was discussed. The topics covered ranged from diagnosis of a medical condition through referral for sperm cryopreservation, the maintenance of the samples in storage, the process of follow-up, and the ultimate fate of frozen samples (use in treatment or disposal). The meeting attracted a multidisciplinary audience of nurses, counselors, scientists, and medical staff from a variety of specialties (e.g. oncology, hematology, fertility), and led for the first time in the UK to a sharing of knowledge on this topic. The workshop demonstrated quite clearly that, despite sperm banks working within the same broad regulatory framework, clinical, counseling and scientific practices varied enormously. There were clearly issues at the boundaries of those disciplines, which were often barriers to providing a joined-up service.

Following the British Andrology Society meeting, feedback from delegates prompted us to write a brief summary so that the spirit of the meeting could be shared more widely. This was published in *Human Fertility* in 2003. However, further feedback suggested that the article did not go far enough and what was needed was a single source of reference for anyone involved in the day-to-day delivery of sperm banking services. Hence the idea for this book was born. For this volume, we have deliberately invited experts in discrete areas of medicine, law, medical, and social science to contribute from within their own field to provide input into the sperm banking process from their own perspectives. We are grateful for their contributions and hope they will accept in good spirit our editing in order to dovetail the various chapters into one another in an attempt to outline the various sperm banking process as a continuum.

Acknowledgements

There are many people to thank in preparing this book. First of all to the staff of Cambridge University Press who kept their belief that we would be able to deliver a final typescript eventually. Primarily, we would like to thank Peter Silver, with whom we first discussed our idea, and then subsequently Betty Fulford, Nicholas Dunton, and Katie James who guided us through the process. Thanks also go to our authors for delivering their chapters but also in allowing us to change them to improve the dovetailing between them throughout the book. We are grateful to Dr. Anthony Hirsch for providing the diagrams for Figures 6.5 and 6.6. Finally, we must acknowledge the support of our respective Heads of Department (Professor William Ledger in Sheffield and Mr. James Hopkisson in Nottingham) for allowing us to engage our time on this project, perhaps to the detriment of other things we should have been doing.

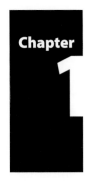

Chapter

1

The history of sperm cryopreservation

Eric M. Walters, James D. Benson, Erik J. Woods, and John K. Critser

Importance of sperm cryopreservation

While there have been several relatively recent comprehensive reviews of mammalian sperm cryopreservation (Watson, 2001; Leibo, 2004), this chapter is not meant to be a review of the literature of mammalian sperm cryopreservation. Instead, we intend to provide an understanding of the history, current status, and potential future direction of mammalian sperm cryobiology. There are many reasons why sperm cryopreservation is important, including: (1) maintenance of genetic diversity in domestic and wild species populations (Wildt, 1992; Critser & Russell, 2000); (2) facilitating the distribution of "genetically superior" domestic species lines; (3) treatment of iatrogenic infertility (Kuczynski et al., 2001; Ranganathan et al., 2002; Tash et al., 2003; Agarwal et al., 2004; Nalesnik et al., 2004); and (4) genetic banking of genetically modified animal models of human health and disease (Critser & Russell, 2000; Knight & Abbott, 2002).

While actual references to sperm cryobiology and cryopreservation date as far back as the 1600s (Sherman, 1964), it was not until the development of artificial insemination (AI) in the late 1950s and early 1960s, when the dairy industry needed longer-term storage methods for bull sperm, that sperm cryopreservation became a major area of scientific investigation. Polge et al. (1949) made a pivotal discovery that showed that the use of glycerol (a permeating solute) could provide protection to cells at low temperatures. This is often cited as the defining moment in the establishment of modern sperm cryobiology. However, there is actually a very important body of literature which predates it, some of which established the scientific basis upon which their work was interpreted and further developed (Lovelock, 1953a; Lovelock & Polge, 1954; Menz & Luyet, 1965; Luyet, 1966; MacKenzie & Luyet, 1967a; 1967b; Luyet & Rapatz, 1970; Luyet, 1971; Rasmussen & Luyet, 1972; Rapatz & Luyet, 1973), and some of which was parallel literature that was not incorporated into the main pathway of sperm cryobiology mainly because it was published in Russian (Katkov, 2005).

Based upon this scientific history, the development of "successful" mammalian sperm cryopresveration methods was established. It is critical to realize, however, that even today only a very few mammalian species' sperm can be effectively cryopreserved. Even in those cases, the "success," as measured by postthaw motility, routinely is 50 percent or less than that of the prefreeze motility. Successful cryopreservation varies highly among species, individuals within species, and even within ejaculates of individuals, which is largely attributed to the differences in biophysical characteristics among cell types (Gao et al., 1997; Thurston et al., 2002; Walters et al., 2005).

Sperm Banking: Theory and Practice, eds. Allan A. Pacey and Mathew J. Tomlinson.
Published by Cambridge University Press. © Cambridge University Press 2009.

History of AI and sperm cryopreservation

It is believed that Lazzaro Spallanzani performed the first successful AI in 1780. Spallanzani inseminated a confined bitch in heat by depositing semen in the uterus with a syringe. This resulted in the birth of three pups 62 days later that resembled the dam as well as the semen donor (Herman, 1981). Other investigators repeated the work of Spallanzani, including John Hunter in 1799, which resulted in a human pregnancy (Herman, 1981). It was not until the 1880s that AI became a means of improving fertility and increasing the number of offspring that one sire could achieve in a lifetime. An English dog breeder between 1884 and 1896 used AI to breed several bitches with one ejaculate (Herman, 1981). At about the same time a French veterinarian demonstrated the effectiveness of AI as a way of improving fertility in the horse as well. Following these initial demonstrations of the effectiveness of AI, horse centers began to spring up all over Europe to collect and extend semen and breed mares (Herman, 1981). The techniques for AI, training of technicians, and improved methods for collection and extending semen continued to increase, and, by 1938, it was reported that some 40000 mares, 1.2 million cows, and 15 million sheep had been serviced by AI in Russia (Herman, 1981).

In the early 1800s most of the AI work was being conducted in Europe or Russia; however, there had been successful attempts at AI in horses and cattle in the USA as well. In 1907 a calf was born from AI by L.L. Lewis at the Oklahoma Experimental Station (Herman, 1981). After this successful AI attempt in cattle, the use of AI in the USA increased, and, in 1937, the practice was started in the dairy herd at the University of Missouri, and, subsequently at other agricultural universities such as Cornell, Minnesota, Nebraska, Wisconsin, and Tennessee (Herman, 1981). In 1939 the American Society of Animal Production (ASAP) was founded by investigators from several universities to discuss and develop protocols for semen collection, evaluation, and preservation from domestic animals, and in particular, the bull (Foote, 1998). It was believed that with the continued development of AI, the dairy industry in the USA could start progressive breeding programs and begin advancing the industry from a genetic perspective. Research programs across the country began investigating sperm biology in terms of collection, equipment, evaluation of sperm morphology, and composition of extenders for both sperm biology and fundamental cryobiology (Foote, 1998).

Cryopreservation of bull sperm

The development of cryopreservation protocols for the bull to be used for AI in the dairy industry began in the 1950s. Bratton et al. (1955) demonstrated in field trials that bovine sperm frozen to −79°C and packed on dry ice could still yield high fertility. Several different media formulations were then investigated in terms of their ability to maintain a high level of motility postthaw at reduced temperatures, and these were termed "extenders." Early in extender development it was found that lipids in egg yolk could protect bull sperm from "cold shock," the sensitivity of cells to reduced temperatures (Watson & Martin, 1973; Watson, 1975; Watson & Martin, 1975; Foote, 1998). The lipid work, in combination with the discovery of the cryoprotective properties of glycerol, aided the development of freezing extenders for cryopreservation of bull sperm. The sum of these discoveries yielded the Tris-egg yolk–glycerol method for freezing bull sperm, which has now become a standard (Foote, 1970; Watson & Martin, 1973; Watson, 1975; Watson & Martin, 1975).

Cryopreservation of boar sperm

Preservation of boar sperm was developed in the 1970s; however, the method used was different than that for other species. Specifically, Pursel & Johnson (1975) developed a "pellet" method for successful freezing of boar sperm. First, samples were cooled to 5 °C at a rate of 0.22 °C/min. At this temperature, cooled media containing extender and glycerol were added. After the addition of glycerol, aliquots of the samples were placed directly on a block of dry ice (−79 °C) and then plunged into liquid nitrogen (−196 °C). This pellet method was relatively effective in terms of postthaw motility, but a major drawback was the inability to label the pellets individually and the difficulty involved with shipment of the samples. In recent years, other methods have been developed such as "maxi" (5 mL) and "mini" (0.25 or 0.5 cc) straws, which allow individual identification and ability to ship domestically and internationally (Bwanga *et al.*, 1990, 1991).

Cryopreservation of mouse sperm

G.L. Rappatz's unpublished and undated work is believed to be the first successful attempt to produce live mice from frozen sperm. In a review by Graham *et al.* (1978) Rappatz's work was discussed as part of a final progress report. However, cryopreservation of mouse sperm was not studied intensively until three independent groups reported successful cryopreservation essentially simultaneously (Okuyama *et al.*, 1990; Tada *et al.*, 1990; Yokoyama *et al.*, 1990). Laboratories across the world have repeated these findings and reported acceptable postthaw viability, but most success has been limited to sperm samples from hybrid or mixed genetic backgrounds (Bath, 2003). Sperm cryopreservation protocols for inbred strains (e.g. C57BL/6) have only been marginally successful due to their extreme sensitivity to the multiple procedural steps involved, such as pipetting, centrifugation, addition and removal of cryoprotective agents (CPAs), and hypothermia (Willoughby *et al.*, 1996; Katkov & Mazur, 1998, 1999; Agca *et al.*, 2002).

There are known differences in terms of fertility and cryosurvival between genotypes of mice (Pomp & Eisen, 1990; Rall *et al.*, 2000) as well as other species such as the rat (Rall *et al.*, 2000) and pig (Thurston *et al.*, 2002). It has been shown that the efficiency of in vitro fertilization (IVF) using fresh sperm is highly variable between genetic backgrounds; for example the fertilization rates (two-cell development) for an inbred line (BALB/c) are lower than fertilization rates for a hybrid line (B6C3F1) (Kawase *et al.*, 2004). Kawase *et al.*, (2004) also reported a difference in the fertilization rates between BALB/c (26 percent) and C57BL/6 (85 percent) for IVF with fresh sperm. The fertilization rates for conventional IVF were even further reduced with frozen–thawed sperm from B6C3F1 males (Kawase *et al.*, 2004). Frozen–thawed sperm from an inbred strain used in a conventional IVF system usually results in very low efficiency largely owing to the lack of motility and cellular damage that occurs during cryopreservation. Futhermore, Nishizono *et al.* (2004) reported that frozen–thawed C57BL/6 sperm had abnormal mitochondrial morphology. In addition, Willoughby *et al.* (1996) reported a significant difference between ICR and B6C3F1 for the percentage of sperm maintaining functional mitochondria following hypo- and hyperosmotic exposure. Nishizono *et al.* (2004) also reported a strain difference between inbred mice, C57BL/6J, and DBA/2N in cryopreservation-induced cellular injury. In the C57BL/6J sperm 83.7 percent of the sperm were damaged compared with DBA/2N (10 percent).

3

Cryopreservation of human sperm

The glycerol work of Polge *et al.* (1949) laid the foundation for cryopreservation of human sperm. In 1953 Sherman and Bunge froze human sperm equilibrated with 10 percent glycerol on dry ice with a 67 percent survival rate. Shortly thereafter Sherman and Bunge (1953) reported three pregnancies with the use of AI in combination with frozen–thawed sperm. After this report of pregnancies following insemination with frozen–thawed cells, many groups began working toward cryopreservation as a treatment for infertility. Sherman continued to pursue the improvement of human sperm preservation by investigating various cryopreservation protocols along with freeze-drying techniques (Sherman, 1954, 1963). One of Sherman's discoveries was that storing human sperm at liquid nitrogen (LN_2) temperature ($-196\,^\circ$C) was superior to storage at $-75\,^\circ$C. In addition, no loss of motility was observed when the sperm were stored in LN_2 for one year; however, there was a decline in motility after storage at $-75\,^\circ$C (Sherman, 1963). Prior to 1964 all pregnancies were produced from short-term storage of sperm; however, Perloff *et al.* (1964) reported pregnancies from insemination with frozen–thawed sperm stored for one to 5.5 months.

History of fundamental cryobiology

Before outlining the history of fundamental cryobiology we must first understand what fundamental cryobiology is and why it falls into a separate category. Cryobiology has functioned for centuries as an observational science. From at least 1787 the effects of cold temperatures on cells have been investigated empirically (Luyet & Gehenio, 1940). Before Polge *et al.* (1949) made their accidental discovery of glycerol as a cryoprotectant (a fortuitous empirical observation), the nascent field had been limited to descriptions of cellular and tissue behavior of many different cell types at subphysiologic temperatures. These empirical studies, however, formed a basis for a theory of the causes of freezing success or failure. The discovery of CPAs opened the doors to a new type of cryobiological study because new variables had been identified that could be used in the optimization of cryopreservation protocols.

In comparison with classic empirical cryobiology, fundamental cryobiology is the quantitative study of the biophysical and biochemical phenomena that occur during cryobiological procedures. These include the transmembrane fluxes associated with the addition and removal of CPAs, the change in chemical potentials during cooling and warming, both intracellular and extracellular ice formation, the effects of cooling and warming rates and storage temperatures, heat transfer in solutions and tissues, and, most importantly, the optimization of cryobiological procedures in conjunction with this information. Because, paradoxically, freezing is used both with the goal of preserving cells and of selectively destroying them, we have been careful to define fundamental cryobiology in the most general context. In the context of this chapter, however, we may be more specific: fundamental cryobiology attempts to quantify the biophysical phenomena that occur during freezing and thawing in order to use this information to develop theoretically optimized cryopreservation protocols. In fact, we will further limit our discussion to the simplest case of single cells frozen and thawed in suspension (e.g. sperm), and we will try to provide both a theoretic and historic background to this area of cryobiology.

With a proper definition in place we can see that fundamental cryobiology covers an enormous range of topics in science, from physics and chemistry to engineering and mathematics, and it is this amalgamation of sciences that appeals to many investigators from these diverse fields. The first quantitative studies of the biophysical effects of cryo-preservation and the use of this knowledge to predict more optimal cryopreservation protocols were explained in Mazur (1963). In his manuscript Mazur examined the connection between a cell's permeability to water and solutes and the freezing rates at which it might be effectively frozen. Mazur notes that, with the knowledge of the biophysical parameters of the cellular membrane, we may significantly narrow the range of empirical research needed to optimize freezing protocols. This reduction in empirical research is perhaps the most significant advantage of quantitative approaches.

In essence, with his paper Mazur formed the basis for much of the work that we call "fundamental cryobiology" today. For example, presently there is a large canon of literature devoted to determining the membrane permeability characteristics of cell types with the purpose of improving cryobiological protocols. These experiments typically determine membrane permeability coefficients by calculating cell volume as a function of time. Devices to determine these coefficients have included stopped flow apparatus (Liu *et al.*, 2002), electronic particle counters such as Coulter Counters (Gilmore *et al.*, 1998), microscope stages designed to allow the perfusion of fluids while keeping the cells in place (either with a porous membrane or by holding with a pipette) (Gao *et al.*, 1996), and several others (McGrath, 1997). These data are then fit with one of several transmembrane flux models to determine the membrane transport coefficients for a specific cell type (see Kleinhans (1998) for a review). Armed with this knowledge, computer simulation can quickly determine which protocols are most likely to provide a successful cryopreservation scheme. We will discuss this in greater detail below. Interestingly, as with many aspects of cryobiology and especially fundamental cryobiology, much research had been done on various cell types before the application of this knowledge to cryopreservation (Jacobs, 1932; Staverman, 1951).

The survival of cells with respect to cooling rate is almost always described in an inverted "U" shape. This may be observed experimentally for many cell types (see Figure 1.1). Mazur's 1962 paper explained quite well that the most probable cause for the second half of the inverted "U" (i.e. higher cooling rates), came from the supercooling (cooling of the solute below its freezing point) induced by cooling at a rate that prevented the cell from maintaining an equilibrium between the intracellular and extracellular milieu. As the cell and the surrounding media cool below freezing, pure water is precipitated out of the extracellular media as ice. This causes an increase in extracellular concentration, which, at slow enough cooling rates, causes the cell to lose water and increase intracellular concentration. When cooling rates are too rapid, water cannot leave the cell quickly enough to maintain equilibrium with the external medium and supercools. Since the probability of ice formation increases with the degree of supercooling (a topic we will discuss in further detail below), the faster the cooling rate the more likely ice will form inside the cell, a major factor of cell death in cryopreservation procedures.

There is considerable debate about the mechanism of damage during slow cooling. Based on the original work of Lovelock (1953a, 1953b), Levitt (1962), and Karow and Webb (1965), Meryman (1968) ascribed the damage of slow cooling to the effects of salt concentrations on human red blood cells and had determined that the membrane became porous to these molecules at extremely high salt concentrations (which are often reached at subzero temperatures). Upon warming the salt molecules were trapped in the membrane, causing a difference in osmotic pressure, an influx of water, and the probable lysis of the cell. Pegg and Diaper (1988) attribute slow cooling injury to decreases in cell volume during slow freezing. In 1972, Mazur and coworkers formalized his explanation of cell damage

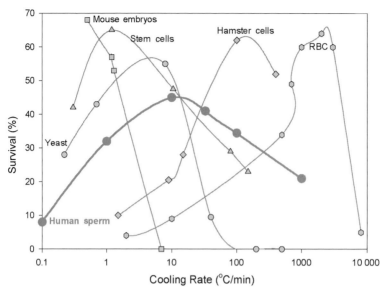

Figure 1.1 Comparison of cryopreservation survival of various cell types as a function of the cooling rate. Note that all cell types shown here demonstrate an inverted "U"-shaped curve, indicating that an ideal cooling rate exists for these cell types. Redrawn and modeled from Mazur (1976).

during freezing and thawing and defined his "two-factor hypothesis" (Mazur *et al.*, 1972). In this manuscript Mazur explained damage at relatively slow cooling rates by the long-term exposure of cells to very high concentrations of non-permeating salts, and damage at relatively high cooling rates by the amount of supercooling that occurs. Regardless of their explanation, both of these damages could be mitigated by the addition of permeating solutes such as glycerol or dimethyl sulfoxide (DMSO). These permeating cryoprotective agents, discovered by Polge *et al.* (1949), had been in use for 25 years, but Mazur's seminal paper gave a much-needed foundation for the development of new cryopreservation protocols and allowed the description of an ideal freezing protocol: cooling just slow enough to avoid more than two degrees of supercooling. After this, a major goal of fundamental cryobiology was to characterize the permeability of the membrane to permeating cryoprotectants, and then use this information to maximize the cooling rate without causing supercooling.

Typically, cryobiologists have dealt with linear cooling rates, most likely because these are the easiest to repeat, calculate in a differential equation, and approximate with cooling apparatus, but the natural cooling rates of objects exposed to low temperatures are exponential (Luyet & Rapatz, 1970). Although there have been several reports of success using non-linear cooling rates (Morris *et al.*, 1999), there was no firm basis for the theory of optimizing non-linear cooling rates until very recently. In 2004, Woelders and Chaveiro (2004) published a theoretical development of non-linear cooling rates developed by fixing the amount of supercooling at two degrees. This allowed them to calculate the cooling rates needed to achieve this fixed amount of supercooling. This, in theory, should be the fastest, "safe," slow cooling rate, but there are many caveats. First, the permeability of the cell to water and solutes must be known at all subzero temperatures. This is not a trivial measurement, and only recently was a method for subzero water permeability measurement published (Devireddy *et al.*, 1998). Additionally, as we will discuss shortly, the probability of ice formation is a function of both supercooling and temperature. Thus there are several variables not accounted for in this model.

Fundamental cryobiology was further advanced in the 1990s by Toner's intracellular ice formation model (Karlsson et al., 1995). This model took into account the temperature, the degree of supercooling, and the cell's inherent ice-nucleating properties to predict a "probability of intracellular ice formation" (P_{IIF}). This P_{IIF} could then be used in conjunction with the Mazur two-factor hypothesis to develop more complicated freezing protocols such as a two-step or three-step protocol where cells were cooled relatively rapidly to a subzero temperature, allowed to equilibrate or partially equilibrate at that temperature, and then cooled rapidly to a plunging temperature (Karlsson et al., 1995; Liu et al., 2000). These protocols allowed investigators to avoid the potentially damaging effects of slowly cooling to zero °C.

Until now, we have mainly discussed the development of "slow" or "equilibrium" cooling protocols. Vitrification, on the other hand, has always been the goal of cryobiologists. Essentially, at high enough cooling rates (>1000°C/min) the extracellular solution does not crystallize, and instead forms an amorphous glass, which is called "vitrification." This vitrification of the solution is associated with little if any cell damage, and is the most appealing cryopreservation protocol because it is so fast (compare this with a standard 1–10°C/min protocol), and has the potential to require no expensive equipment (i.e. plunge the sample directly into LN_2). The downside to vitrification procedures is that although isotonic saline is theoretically vitrifiable, the cooling rates needed to achieve vitrification are on the order of 10^5–10^6°C/min. Alternatively, much work has been done investigating the vitrification properties of many different solutions (Fahy et al., 2004). At higher concentrations, greater than four or five molar, typical CPAs such as glycerol or propylene glycol become vitrifiable at cooling rates of the order of 10^3°C/min.

Unfortunately, as appealing as vitrification seems, there are several downsides. First, the cooling rates are difficult to achieve. In order to achieve ultra-rapid cooling rates, the surface area to volume ratio of the cell suspension (i.e. the container that holds the cells and their suspending solute) must be very high. This has been achieved by use of a "cryo-loop" (Lane et al., 1999). The idea of the cryo-loop is to have a very thin film of solution that maximizes the surface exposed to liquid nitrogen. Alternatively, very thin straws also have a very high surface to volume ratio and have been used successfully to vitrify oocytes (Ramezani et al., 2005). The second problem is achieving the high molar concentrations (4–5M) of permeating cryoprotectants. Many cell types have limits to which they can shrink or swell without significant damage. These limits are called "osmotic tolerance limits" and are cell type and species (sometimes even interspecies) dependent (Walters et al., 2005). For example, Gilmore et al. (1998) established that, when boar sperm swell above 103 percent of their isosmotic volume or shrink below 97 percent of their isosmotic volume, their motility significantly declines. Because the addition of CPAs causes cells to shrink and then re-swell, there is a possibility of adding CPAs in such a way as to cause significant damage to the cell. This consideration is also important while removing CPAs after thawing. Therefore CPA addition and removal protocols, especially in the context of vitrification, often consist of multiple steps. For example, in order to add 1M glycerol to boar sperm, the sperm must first be equilibrated with 0.3M for six seconds, followed by a 0.6M step for another six seconds, a 0.95M step for six seconds, and finally a 1M step. In order to reach remotely vitrifiable concentrations (4M), we would have to perform at least eight steps (see Figure 1.2).

With all of this as background, we will conclude by outlining the typical fundamental cryobiological experiment in the following steps (examples of these experiments may be

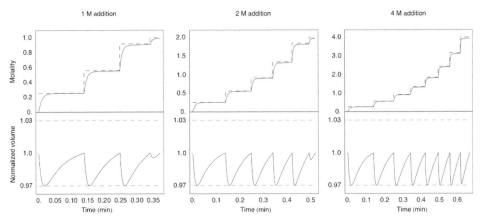

Figure 1.2 Plot of volume and molarity versus time for the addition of glycerol to boar sperm. The dashed lines indicate osmotic tolerance limits (OTLs) and extracellular molality in their respective rows and the solid lines indicate normalized cell volume and intracellular concentration, respectively.

found in Gilmore *et al.*, 1996, 1998; Pfaff *et al.*, 1998; Liu *et al.*, 2000; Woods *et al.*, 2000; Agca *et al.*, 2002; Chaveiro *et al.*, 2004). First, cells are exposed to various anisosmotic salt solutions and their subsequent volume is measured. The reciprocal of concentration versus normalized volume is plotted. This is to establish that cell volume corresponds linearly with a change in osmotic pressure (i.e. they behave as linear or ideal osmometers, the Boyle–Van't Hoff relationship). The intercept of the regression (toward a theoretical infinite concentration) predicts the osmotically inactive fraction of the cell, which is the cell membrane, organelles, proteins, and bound water that will not cross the plasma membrane. This establishes the osmotically inactive portion of the cell (often referred to as V_b). In the case of mammalian sperm this value is usually between 60 and 70 percent of the isosmotic volume (Gilmore *et al.*, 1996; Karow & Critser, 1997; Guthrie *et al.*, 2002).

The next step is to establish the biophysical parameters of solute and water permeability, usually indicated as P_s and L_p, respectively, at several temperatures. Because sperm have an enormous surface area to volume ratio, their permeability is very high relative to other cell types. This poses a significant challenge to the researcher attempting to determine these parameters. This challenge has been surmounted in two different ways. The first and most common has been the use of the Coulter Counter, which records electric pulses proportional to cell volume. This allows the real-time measurement of thousands of cells exposed to various solutions. The second method is the use of a stopped flow apparatus that takes advantage of the relationship between average population volume and light refraction. The advantage of the stopped flow apparatus is its temporal resolution. The disadvantage of the stopped flow apparatus is that the measurement of volume is indirect.

If the experiment were to stop here, we would have enough information to predict both an optimal CPA addition and removal protocol and a probable optimal cooling rate. Alternatively, we can also establish the parameters of the intracellular ice formation model of Karlsson *et al.* (1993). This is done by monitoring cells under a microscope while cooling and noting the percentage of cells which freeze intracellularly at a given temperature and degree of supercooling. After these parameters are established a theoretically optimized protocol can be developed which obeys the fundamental principles outlined in Mazur *et al.* (1972): the optimal freezing protocol cools the cell the fastest while avoiding a degree of supercooling associated with a high probability of ice formation.

Although there is a large amount of work involved in establishing these cryobiological parameters, the work is quite significantly less than that which would be involved in developing a cryopreservation protocol entirely empirically, given the wide variation in cryopreservation protocols. Fundamental cryobiology can give investigators a much narrower band of possibility for empirical experimentation, saving valuable time and resources.

Current state of the art in sperm cryopreservation

Successful sperm cryopreservation requires maintaining the postthaw structural and functional integrity. However, to maintain functional integrity, the compartments of the sperm need to be fully protected so that frozen–thawed sperm can undergo normal fertilization under either in vitro or in vivo conditions. Differences in the various sperm compartments: we expect that each compartment (i.e. acrosome, flagella, midpiece) of sperm will be affected by cryopreservation differently. While motility may be protected at a high level, acrosome integrity may be severely damaged under a similar physical alteration such as osmotic stress (Willoughby et al., 1996; Agca et al., 2002; Guthrie et al., 2002; Walters et al., 2005). Although the effects of an entire cryopreservation procedure on acrosome integrity have been investigated to some extent (Okada et al., 2001; Hollinshead et al., 2003), the specific effects of anisosmotic stress on acrosome integrity have not been previously investigated. Previous investigations have shown that mammalian sperm have a very broad range of osmotic tolerance, as assessed by plasma membrane integrity and motility following exposure to various anisosmotic conditions (Willoughby et al., 1996; Songsasen & Leibo, 1997; Agca et al., 2002).

The methods of cryopreservation of bull sperm have not changed much in the past few years. Recently, there has been some work on the addition of cholesterol to the membrane of bull sperm prior to cryopreservation. Work by Purdy and Graham (2004) has shown that the addition of cholesterol to the membrane improves postthaw motility. In addition, cholesterol added to the membrane did not inhibit fertility, the ability of the sperm to undergo the capacitation, or acrosome reaction. Work is also being done to improve the methodology for cryopreservation; however, it appears currently that the methods are equal to, but not improved over, current systems.

Currently, methods are being developed to freeze boar sperm by alterations of the freezing medium composition such as the addition of antioxidants (Funahashi & Sano, 2005), various forms of packaging the semen for cryopreservation, and freeze-drying. Recently, there has been an effort to investigate the effects of reactive oxygen species on cryopreservation of boar sperm by the addition of antioxidants to the extender prior to freezing. In addition to antioxidants, work is being conducted to determine the effects of the vessel (0.5 cc and 5 mL straws, bags, cryovials) used to freeze boar sperm. In the swine industry, producers will limit the use of frozen–thawed semen if they have to thaw 10–15 0.5 cc straws to achieve the desired AI dose. However, if the producer can thaw one flatpack (containing 5 mL of sperm) and dilute to achieve an AI dose, frozen–thawed boar sperm will have a huge impact on the industry.

An alternative method of preserving pig sperm is freeze-drying, which has the advantage of room temperature storage, but freeze-dried sperm must be used in combination with intra cytoplasmic sperm injection (ICSI), as a high percentage of motility is lost (Kwon et al., 2004). Currently, the biggest drawback to freeze-dried sperm is the low evidence of ICSI-derived offspring in the pig. However, because of the appeal of convenient storage there are many groups currently working in this direction.

9

In the mouse, several alterative methods to traditional cryopreservation protocols have been investigated, such as freeze-drying (Kawase *et al.*, 2005) and cryopreservation without cryoprotectants (Van Thuan *et al.*, 2005). One reason for the large number of methods to freeze mouse sperm is the development and success of many assisted reproductive technologies such as IVF and ICSI. More importantly, the development of ICSI in the mouse has increased the use of frozen–thawed sperm because the postthaw motility does not have to be good. Several groups have begun to gain an understanding of the biophysical and biochemical characteristics of mammalian sperm, which is critical to the development and optimization of strain-specific cryopreservation protocols. Mathematical modeling of these protocols may then be used to determine the optimal addition and removal of CPAs as well as cooling and warming rates for mouse sperm. Fundamental cryobiological properties associated with osmotic changes such as the membrane permeability to water (L_p) and cryoprotectants (P_s), their activation energies (E_a), and the sperm's osmotic tolerance limits (OTL) (Willoughby *et al.*, 1996) are critical to the development of cryopreservation protocols. Walters *et al.* (2005) investigated the OTLs of mouse sperm from various genetic backgrounds for maintenance of motility, plasma membrane, and acrosomal integrity, and found that maintenance of motility was affected by the genetic background; however, plasma membrane and acrosomal integrity were not. With the OTLs as well as some of the other cryobiological parameters of mouse sperm from different genetic backgrounds we can begin to provide the fundamental basis for the development of species and even strain-specific cryopreservation protocols.

Cryopreservation of human sperm has been developed for many different reasons, including development of assisted reproductive technologies such as intracytoplasmic sperm injection, "fertility insurance" for potential illness-induced infertility early in childhood, and azoospermic patients. As an example of "fertility insurance," Horne *et al.* (2004) have reported the birth of a live offspring utilizing IVF/ICSI with sperm that had been cryopreserved for 21 years (see Chapter 8). The postthaw motility of human sperm can range from 20 percent to 50 percent (Sbracia *et al.*, 1997). This loss of motility of human sperm after cryopreservation is believed to be caused by several factors, including diminished integrity of the membranes and cryodamage to the membranes of the intracellular compartments, which then affects energy metabolism and synthesis. Early work by Critser *et al.* (1987a, 1987b) also showed that loss of motility is largely caused by the addition and removal of CPAs, which cause the sperm to shrink and swell beyond their OTLs. Additionally, there has been work investigating the addition of components such as hyaluronan, a polysaccharide which mediates cell locomotion (Laurent, 1987) to the postthaw medium to increase postthaw motility. Sbracia *et al.* (1997) added sodium hyaluronate to the postthaw medium, which improved postthaw motility at 30 minutes postthaw. However, 24 hours after thawing there was no difference in motility between control and treated sperm.

Applications of sperm cryopreservation

Human semen cryopreservation for iatrogenic infertility

Over the last few decades there have been many improvements to human medicine that have greatly increased the indications for sperm banking. This will be discussed in more detail in later chapters of this book. However, briefly, the many advances achieved in cancer therapies for men of pediatric, adolescent, and reproductive age have led to increases in long-term survival, making posttreatment quality of life increasingly important and deserving of more attention. Specifically, surgery, radiation therapy, and chemotherapy may achieve relatively high remission rates in patients with cancers such as seminoma, yet can be very detrimental to male fertility and therefore preclude these survivors from having genetically related children. Surgery may result in mechanical insult directly to the gonad, its innervations, and its vascularity, while radiation and chemotherapy both compromise fertility through cytotoxic effects – the degree of which is based on the regimen used and the duration of the treatment (see Chapter 2). Additionally, fertility can be impaired indirectly through injury to the hypothalamus or pituitary glands, causing secondary hypogonadism (Puscheck et al., 2004). In these individuals, posttreatment, some degree of fertility may return; however, who will recover fertility and to what degree cannot be predicted. Indeed, the incidence of azoospermia in men after treatment is high, and only 20 percent to 50 percent of these men eventually recover spermatogenesis (Carson et al., 1991). The current method for preserving male fertility for individuals who are at risk of losing it iatrogenically is through cryopreservation of sperm prior to treatment, followed by assisted reproductive techniques (ARTs) at a later date (see Chapter 8).

Non-cancerous, non-testicular-related diseases can also require the use of cytotoxic drugs and immunosuppressive therapies that can permanently suppress spermatogenesis (Ranganathan et al., 2002). They may also include autoimmune disorders and diseases requiring organ transplants. Cryopreservation of sperm prior to these therapies is a viable method for retaining fertility; even if the pretreatment sperm quality is relatively low, enough can usually be recovered for IVF or ICSI.

Sperm cryopreservation may also be indicated to assist in non-cancer-related male infertility. For example storage, pooling, and concentration of many oligozoospermic samples from one male may be used to increase the total number of cells for intrauterine insemination (IUI) or IVF (Kuczynski et al., 2001). Cryopreservation is also beneficial in this case in the event of unexpected azoospermia on the day of the procedure, or inability to produce a sample if insemination with a fresh sample is to be attempted (Anger et al., 2003). This will be discussed in more detail in later chapters.

If a male elects for corrective surgical treatment for a reproductive problem, cryopreservation prior to the procedure may be of benefit as well. This could include surgeries such as varicocele ligation for oligozoospermia as an insurance against postsurgical azoospermia due to recurrent varicocele, hydrocele, or injury to the testis during the surgery (Anger et al., 2003). Likewise, sperm may be cryopreserved prior to planned transurethral resection of the ejaculatory ducts (TURED) by first harvesting sperm via seminal vesicle aspiration from men undergoing this surgery for oligozoospermia, azoospermia, or pain due to ejaculatory duct obstruction.

Cryopreservation of sperm from critically ill or deceased men

Postmortem sperm retrieval (PMSR) is technically feasible following brain death with respirator maintenance or within 24 hours of death without a respirator, using vasal aspiration or epididymal/testicular retrieval (Tash et al., 2003). Although technically possible, the retrieval and use of sperm from dying or deceased men is fraught with ethical and legal ramifications (see Chapter 5). Additionally, sperm production can be profoundly impaired during a terminal illness. This may not only make recovery difficult but may also make successful cryopreservation and recovery of motile sperm impossible. It will ultimately be up to the practitioner to ensure that institutional guidelines, which take into account the legal climate of the region, are in place and followed before proceeding with attempts at PMSR.

Genetic banking of laboratory animal models of human health and disease

During the past several years the use of genetically engineered animal models (GEMs), which have been widely used for understanding human diseases, has increased exponentially (Knight & Abbott, 2002). This increase has been so momentous that the ability to maintain these animals has become unrealistic (Sharp & Mobraaten, 1997; Knight & Abbott, 2002). The number of males needed to create a sperm bank of GEM lines would be significantly less than the number of females needed to create a similar embryo bank. Although current cryobanking methods of embryos from these lines has been the main means of genome banking, the number of animals needed to produce adequate numbers of embryos presents a significant drawback (Whittingham, 1974; Rall et al., 2000). On the other hand, sperm banking is only appropriate when preserving the haploid genome is satisfactory (Critser & Mobraaten, 2000; Nakagata, 2000). The ability to cryopreserve mammalian sperm would significantly alleviate much of the strain on research animal infrastructure related to housing GEM lines by providing a cost-effective and efficient storage approach (Thornton et al., 1999; Glenister & Thornton, 2000). In addition, sperm cryopreservation in combination with ARTs such as AI, IVF, and ICSI procedures could greatly facilitate rederivation of GEM (Thornton et al., 1999). ICSI is technically a very demanding ART and requires high set-up costs; however, it can allow the utilization of frozen–thawed sperm with low-motility or damaged sperm. With the development of ICSI there is continued need for the development and understanding of fundamental cryobiology parameters to enhance the ability to preserve sperm from endangered species and GEMs.

Conclusion

The history of mammalian sperm cryopreservation dates back several centuries to when the motility of sperm cooled by snow was measured (Sherman, 1964). We have made great progress in sperm cryopreservation, as the sperm of many species have been successfully cryopreserved with resulting offspring. However, there are still many avenues that need to be explored as ARTs in different species become available and cryopreservation efficiencies improve. Furthermore, the possible applications of sperm cryopreservation continue to increase as new GEM models are developed for the understanding of many human diseases. The future of sperm cryopreservation continues to have a positive outlook.

References

Agarwal, A., Ranganathan, P., Kattal, N. et al. (2004). Fertility after cancer: a prospective review of assisted reproductive outcome with banked semen specimens. Fertility and Sterility, 81, 342–8.

Agca, Y., Gilmore, J., Byers, M. et al. (2002). Osmotic characteristics of mouse spermato-zoa in the presence of extenders and sugars. Biology of Reproduction, 67, 1493–1501.

Anger, J.T., Gilbert, B.R. & Goldstein, M. (2003). Cryopreservation of sperm: indications, methods and results. Journal of Urology, 170, 1079–84.

Bath, M.L. (2003). Simple and efficient in vitro fertilization with cryopreserved C57BL/6J mouse sperm. Biology of Reproduction, 68, 19–23.

Bratton, R.W., Foote, R.H. & Cruthers, J.C. (1955). Preliminary fertility results with frozen bovine spermatozoa. *Journal of Dairy Science*, **38**, 40–6.

Bwanga, C.O., de Braganca, M.M., Einarsson, S. & Rodriguez-Martinez, H. (1990). Cryopreservation of boar semen in mini- and maxi-straws. *Zentralblatt für Veterinärmedizin Reihe A*, **37**, 651–8.

Bwanga, C.O., Hofmo, P.O., Grevle, I.S., Einarsson, S. & Rodriguez-Martinez, H. (1991). In vivo fertilizing capacity of deep frozen boar semen packaged in plastic bags and maxi-straws. *Zentralblatt für Veterinärmedizin Reihe A*, **38**, 281–6.

Carson, S.A., Smith, A.L., Scoggan, J.L. & Buster, J.E. (1991). Superovulation fails to increase human blastocyst yield after uterine lavage. *Prenatal Diagnosis*, **11**, 513–22.

Chaveiro, A., Liu, J., Mullen, S., Woelders, H. & Critser, J.K. (2004). Determination of bull sperm membrane permeability to water and cryoprotectants using a concentration-dependent self-quenching fluorophore. *Cryobiology*, **48**, 72–80.

Critser, J.K. & Mobraaten, L.E. (2000). Cryopreservation of murine spermatozoa. *Institute of Laboratory Animal Research Journal*, **41**, 197–206.

Critser, J.K. & Russell, R.J. (2000). Genome resource banking of laboratory animal models. *Institute of Laboratory Animal Research Journal*, **41**, 183–6.

Critser, J.K., Huse-Benda, A.R., Aaker, D.V., Arneson, B.W. & Ball, G.D. (1987a). Cryopreservation of human spermatozoa. I. Effects of holding procedure and seeding on motility, fertilizability, and acrosome reaction. *Fertility and Sterility*, **47**, 656–63.

Critser, J.K., Arneson, B.W., Aaker, D.V., Huse-Benda, A.R. & Ball, G.D. (1987b). Cryopreservation of human spermatozoa. II. Post-thaw chronology of motility and of zona-free hamster ova penetration. *Fertility and Sterility*, **47**, 980–4.

Devireddy, R.V., Raha, D. & Bischof, J.C. (1998). Measurement of water transport during freezing in cell suspensions using a differential scanning calorimeter. *Cryobiology*, **36**, 124–55.

Fahy, G.M., Wowk, B., Wu, J. *et al.* (2004). Cryopreservation of organs by vitrification: perspectives and recent advances. *Cryobiology*, **48**, 157–78.

Foote, R.H. (1970). Influence of extender, extension rate, and glycerolating technique on fertility of frozen bull semen. *Journal of Dairy Science*, **53**, 1478–82.

Foote, R.H. (1998). *Artificial Insemination to Cloning: Tracing 50 Years of Research*. Ithaca, NY: New York State College of Agriculture & Life.

Funahashi, H. & Sano, T. (2005). Select antioxidants improve the function of extended boar semen stored at 10 degrees C. *Theriogenology*, **63**, 1605–16.

Gao, D.Y., Benson, C.T., Liu, C. *et al.* (1996). Development of a novel microperfusion chamber for determination of cell membrane transport properties. *Biophysical Journal*, **71**, 443–50.

Gao, D., Mazur, P. & Critser, J.K. (1997). Fundamental cryobiology of mammalian spermatozoa. In A.M. Karow and J.K. Critser, eds., *Reproductive Tissue Banking; Scientific Principles*. San Diego, CA: Academic Press, pp. 263–313.

Gilmore, J.A., Du, J., Tao, J., Peter, A.T. & Critser, J.K. (1996). Osmotic properties of boar spermatozoa and their relevance to cryopreservation. *Journal of Reproduction and Fertility*, **107**, 87–95.

Gilmore, J.A., Liu, J., Peter, A.T. & Critser, J.K. (1998). Determination of plasma membrane characteristics of boar spermatozoa and their relevance to cryopreservation. *Biology of Reproduction*, **58**, 28–36.

Glenister, P.H. & Thornton, C.E. (2000). Cryoconservation-archiving for the future. *Mammalian Genome*, **11**, 565–71.

Graham, E.F., Crabo, B.G. & Pace, M.M. (1978). Current status of semen preservation in the ram, boar and stallion. *Journal of Animal Science*, **47**, 80–119.

Guthrie, H.D., Liu, J. & Critser, J.K. (2002). Osmotic tolerance limits and effects of cryoprotectants on motility of bovine spermatozoa. *Biology of Reproduction*, **67**, 1811–16.

Herman, H. (1981). *Improving Cattle by the Millions*. Columbia, MO: University of Missouri Press.

Hollinshead, F.K., Gillan, L., O'Brien, J.K., Evans, G. & Maxwell, W.M. (2003). In vitro and in vivo assessment of functional capacity of flow cytometrically sorted ram spermatozoa after freezing and thawing. *Reproduction Fertility and Development*, **15**, 351–9.

Horne, G., Atkinson, A.D., Pease, E.H. *et al.* (2004). Live birth with sperm cryopreserved for 21 years prior to cancer treatment: case report. *Human Reproduction*, **19**, 1448–9.

Jacobs, M.H. (1932). The simultaneous measurement of cell permeability to water and dissolved substances. *Journal of Cellular and Comparative Physiology*, **2**, 427–44.

Karlsson, J.O.M., Cravalho, E.G. & Toner, M. (1993). Intracellular ice formation: causes and consequences. *Cryoletters*, **14**, 323–36.

Karlsson, J.O.M., Eroglu, A., Toth, T.L., Cravalho, E.G. & Toner, M. (1995). Rational design and theoretical optimization of a cryopreservation protocol. In: *Proceedings of the 1995 ASME International Mechanical Engineering Congress and Exposition. San Francisco, CA, USA: Advances in Heat Mass Transfer in Biotechnology, American Society of Mechanical Engineers, Heat Transfer Division, (Publication) HTD. v 322.* New York, NY: ASME.

Karow, A.M. & Critser, J.K. (1997). *Reproductive Tissue Banking: Scientific Principles*. San Diego, CA: Academic Press.

Karow, A.M. Jr, & Webb W.R. (1965). Tissue freezing. A theory for injury and survival. *Cryobiology*, **2**, 99–108.

Katkov, I.I. (2005). Exact solution for the time of maximum volume excursion. 2-solute systems. *Cryobiology*, **51**, 384.

Katkov, I.I. & Mazur, P. (1998). Influence of centrifugation regimes on motility, yield, and cell associations of mouse spermatozoa. *Journal of Andrology*, **19**, 232–41.

Katkov, I.I. & Mazur, P. (1999). Factors affecting yield and survival of cells when suspensions are subjected to centrifugation. Influence of centrifugal acceleration, time of centrifugation, and length of the suspension column in quasi-homogeneous centrifugal fields. *Cell Biochemistry and Biophysics*, **31**, 231–45.

Kawase, Y., Aoki, Y., Kamada, N., Jishage, K. & Suzuki, H. (2004). Comparison of fertility between intracytoplasmic sperm injection and in vitro fertilization with a partial zona pellucida incision by using a piezo-micromanipulator in cryopreserved inbred mouse spermatozoa. *Contemporary Topics in Laboratory Animal Science*, **43**, 21–5.

Kawase, Y., Araya, H., Kamada, N., Jishage, K. & Suzuki, H. (2005). Possibility of long-term preservation of freeze-dried mouse spermatozoa. *Biology of Reproduction*, **72**, 568–73.

Kleinhans, F.W. (1998). Membrane permeability modeling: Kedem-Katchalsky vs a two-parameter formalism. *Cryobiology*, **37**, 271–89.

Knight, J. & Abbott, A. (2002). Full house. *Nature*, **417**, 785–6.

Kuczynski, W., Dhont, M., Grygoruk, C. *et al.* (2001). The outcome of intracytoplasmic injection of fresh and cryopreserved ejaculated spermatozoa – a prospective randomized study. *Human Reproduction*, **16**, 2109–13.

Kwon, I.K., Park, K.E. & Niwa, K. (2004). Activation, pronuclear formation, and development in vitro of pig oocytes following intracytoplasmic injection of freeze-dried spermatozoa. *Biology of Reproduction*, **71**, 1430–36.

Lane, M., Schoolcraft, W.B. & Gardner, D.K. (1999). Vitrification of mouse and human blastocysts using a novel cryoloop container-less technique. *Fertility and Sterility*, **72**, 1073–8.

Leibo, S.P. (2004). *The Early History of Gamete Cryobiology. Life in the Frozen State*, eds. B. Fuller, N. Lane & E.E. Benson. Boca Raton, FL: CRC Press.

Levitt, J. (1962). A sulfhydryl disulphide hypothesis of frost injury and resistance in plants. *Journal of Theoretical Biology*, **3**, 355.

Liu, J., Woods, E.J., Agca, Y., Critser, E.S. & Critser, J.K. (2000). Cryobiology of rat embryos II: A theoretical model for the development of interrupted slow freezing procedures. *Biology of Reproduction*, **63**, 1303–12.

Liu, J. Christian, J.A. & Critser, J.K. (2002). Canine RBC osmotic tolerance and membrane permeability. *Cryobiology*, **44**, 258–68.

Lovelock, J.E. (1953a). The haemolysis of human red blood-cells by freezing and thawing. *Biochimica et Biophysica Acta*, **10**, 414–26.

Lovelock, J.E. (1953b). The mechanism of the protective action of glycerol against haemolysis by freezing and thawing. *Biochimica et Biophysica Acta*, **11**, 28–36.

Lovelock, J.E. & Polge, C. (1954). The immobilization of spermatozoa by freezing and thawing and the protective action of glycerol. *Biochemical Journal*, **58**, 618–22.

Luyet, B.J. (1966). Notes on the coordination of basic research in cryobiology and of applied research in the cryopreservation of organs and organized tissues, with particular reference to skin. *Cryobiology*, **3**, 97–108.

Luyet, B & Gehenio, P. (1940). *Life and Death at Low Temperatures*. Normandy, MO: Biodynamica.

Luyet, B, & Rapatz, G. (1970). A review of basic researches on the cryopreservation of red blood cells. *Cryobiology*, **6**, 425–82.

MacKenzie, A.P. & Luyet, B.J. (1967a). Electron microscope study of recrystallization in rapidly frozen gelatin gels. *Biodynamica*, **10**, 95–122.

MacKenzie, A.P. & Luyet, B.J. (1967b). Freeze-drying and protein denaturation in muscle tissue; losses in protein solubility. *Nature*, **215**, 83–4.

Mazur, P. (1963). Kinetics of water loss from cells at subzero temperatures and the likelihood of intracellular freezing. *Journal of General Physiology*, **47**, 347–69.

Mazur, P. (1976). Freezing and low temperature storage of living cells. In O. Muhlbock, ed., *Proceedings of the Workshop on Basic Aspects of Freeze Preservation of Mouse Strains*. Bar Harbor, FL: Jackson Laboratory, pp. 1–12.

Mazur, P., Leibo, S.P. & Chu, E.H. (1972). A two-factor hypothesis of freezing injury. Evidence from Chinese hamster tissue-culture cells. *Experimental Cell Research*, **71**, 345–55.

McGrath, J.J. (1997). Quantitative measurement of cell membrane transport: technology and applications. *Cryobiology*, **34**, 315–34.

Menz, L.J. & Luyet, B.J. (1965). A study of the lines of fracture observed in the freeze-drying of aqueous solutions crystallized into spherulites. *Biodynamica*, **9**, 265–75.

Menz, L. & Luyet, B. (1971). Electron microscope study of rapidly frozen suspensions of leucocytes. *Biodynamica*, **11**, 59–68.

Meryman, H.T. (1968). Modified model for the mechanism of freezing injury in erythrocytes. *Nature*, **218**, 333–6.

Morris, G.J., Acton, E. & Avery, S. (1999). A novel approach to sperm cryopreservation. *Human Reproduction*, **14**, 1013–21.

Nakagata, N. (2000). Cryopreservation of mouse spermatozoa. *Mammalian Genome*, **11**, 572–6.

Nalesnik, J.G., Sabanegh, E.S. Jr., Eng, T.Y. & Buchholz, T.A. (2004). Fertility in men after treatment for stage 1 and 2A seminoma. *American Journal of Clinical Oncology*, **27**, 584–8.

Nishizono, H., Shioda, M., Takeo, T., Irie, T. & Nakagata, N. (2004). Decrease of fertilizing ability of mouse spermatozoa after freezing and thawing is related to cellular injury. *Biology of Reproduction*, **71**, 973–8.

Okada, A., Igarashi, H., Kuroda, M. *et al.* (2001). Cryopreservation-induced acrosomal vesiculation in live spermatozoa from cynomolgus monkeys (*Macaca fascicularis*). *Human Reproduction*, **16**, 2139–47.

Okuyama, M., Isogai, S., Hamada, H. & Ogawa, S. (1990). In vitro fertilization (IVF) and artificial insemination (AI) by cryopreserved spermatozoa in the mouse. *Journal of Fertility and Implantation*, **7**, 116–19.

Pegg, D.E. & Diaper, M.P. (1988). On the mechanism of injury to slowly frozen erythrocytes. *Biophysical Journal*, **54**, 471–88.

Perloff, W.H., Steinberger, E. & Sherman, J.K. (1964). Conception with human spermatozoa frozen by nitrogen vapor technic. *Fertility and Sterility*, **25**, 501–4.

Pfaff, R.T., Liu, J., Gao, D. *et al.* (1998). Water and DMSO membrane permeability characteristics of in vivo and in vitro-derived and cultured murine oocytes and embryos. *Molecular Human Reproduction*, **4**, 51–9.

Polge, C., Smith, A. & Parkes, A. (1949). Revival of spermatozoa after vitrification and dehydration at low temperatures. *Nature*, **164**, 666.

Pomp, D. & Eisen, E.J. (1990). Genetic control of survival of frozen mouse embryos. *Biology of Reproduction*, **42**, 775–86.

Purdy, P.H. & Graham, J.K. (2004). Effect of adding cholesterol to bull sperm membranes on sperm capacitation, the acrosome reaction, and fertility. *Biology of Reproduction*, **71**, 522–7.

Pursel, V.G. & Johnson, L.A. (1975). Freezing of boar spermatozoa: fertilizing capacity with concentrated semen and a new thawing procedure. *Journal of Animal Science*, **40**, 99–102.

Puscheck, E., Philip, P.A. & Jeyendran, R.S. (2004). Male fertility preservation and cancer treatment. *Cancer Treatment Reviews*, **30**, 173–80.

Rall, W. F, Schmidt, P.M., Lin, X. *et al.* (2000). Factors affecting the efficiency of embryo cryopreservation and rederivation of rat and mouse models. *Institute of Laboratory Animal Research Journal*, **41**, 221–7.

Ramezani, M., Valojerdi, M.R. & Parivar, K. (2005). Effect of three vitrification methods on development of two-cell mouse embryos. *CryoLetters*, **26**, 85–92.

Ranganathan, P., Mahran, A.M., Hallak, J. & Agarwal, A. (2002). Sperm cryopreservation for men with nonmalignant, systemic diseases: a descriptive study. *Journal of Andrology*, **23**, 71–5.

Rapatz, G. & Luyet, B. (1973). The cryopreservation of blood by the method of two-step freezing. *Biodynamica*, **11**, 169–79.

Rasmussen, D.H. & Luyet, B. (1972). Thermal analysis of "partially dehydrated" heart tissue. *Biodynamica*, **11**, 149–55.

Sbracia, M., Grasso, J., Sayme, N., Stronk, J. & Huszar, G. (1997). Hyaluronic acid substantially increases the retention of motility in cryopreserved/thawed human spermatozoa. *Human Reproduction*, **12**, 1949–54.

Sharp, J. & Mobraaten L. (1997). To save or not to save: the role of repositories in a period of rapidly expanding development of genetically engineered strains of mice. In L.M. Houdebine, ed., *Transgenic Animals: Generation and Use*. Boca Raton, FL: CRC Press, pp. 525–32.

Sherman, J.K. (1954). Freezing and freeze-drying of human spermatozoa. *Fertility and Sterility*, **5**, 357–71.

Sherman, J.K. (1963). Improved methods of preservation of human spermatozoa by freezing and freeze-drying. *Fertility and Sterility*, **14**, 49–64.

Sherman, J.K. (1964). Research on frozen human sperm. In *20th Annual Meeting of the American Society for the Study of Sterility*. Bal Harbour, FL.

Sherman, J.K. & Bunge, R.G. (1953). Observations on preservation of human spermatozoa at low temperatures. *Proceedings of the Society for Experimental Biology and Medicine. Society for Experimental Biology and Medicine*, **82**, 686–8.

Songsasen, N, & Leibo, S.P. (1997). Cryopreservation of mouse spermatozoa. II. Relationship between survival after cryopreservation and osmotic tolerance of spermatozoa from three strains of mice. *Cryobiology*, **35**, 255–69.

Staverman, A. (1951). The theory of measurement of osmotic pressure. *Recueil des Travaux Chimiques des Pays-Bas*, **70**, 344–52.

Tada, N., Sato, M., Yamanoi, J. et al. (1990). Cryopreservation of mouse spermatozoa in the presence of raffinose and glycerol. *Journal of Reproduction and Fertility*, **89**, 511–16.

Tash, J.A., Applegarth, L.D., Kerr, S.M., Fins, J.J., Rosenwaks, Z., & Schlegel, P.N. (2003). Postmortem sperm retrieval: the effect of instituting guidelines. *Journal of Urology*, **170**, 1922–5.

Thornton, C.E., Brown, S.D. & Glenister, P.H. (1999). Large numbers of mice established by in vitro fertilization with cryopreserved spermatozoa: implications and applications for genetic resource banks, mutagenesis screens, and mouse backcrosses. *Mammalian Genome*, **10**, 987–92.

Thurston, L.M., Watson, P.F. & Holt, W.V. (2002). Semen cryopreservation: a genetic explanation for species and individual variation? *CryoLetters*, **23**, 255–62.

Laurent, T.C. (1987). Biochemistry for hyaluronan. *Acta Oto-laryngologica Supplementum*, **442**, 7–24.

Van Thuan, N., Wakayama, S., Kishigami, S. & Wakayama, T. (2005). New preservation method for mouse spermatozoa without freezing. *Biology of Reproduction*, **72**, 444–50.

Walters, E.M., Men, H., Agca, Y. et al. (2005). Osmotic tolerance of mouse spermatozoa from various genetic backgrounds: acrosome integrity, membrane integrity, and maintenance of motility. *Cryobiology*, **50**, 193–205.

Watson, P.F. (1975). The interaction of egg yolk and ram spermatozoa studied with a fluorescent probe. *Journal of Reproduction and Fertility*, **42**, 105–11.

Watson, P.F. (2001). Cryobanking the Genetic Resource. In F. Watson, B. Holt & W.V. Holt, eds., *Vertebrate Germplasm Resource Banking: Strategies and Techniques*. Boca Raton, FL: CRC Press.

Watson, P.F. & Martin, I.C. (1973). The response of ram spermatozoa to preparations of egg yolk in semen diluents during storage at 5 or −196 degrees C. *Australian Journal of Biological Sciences*, **26**, 927–35.

Watson, P.F. & Martin, I.C. (1975). Effects of egg yolk, glycerol and the freezing rate on the viability and acrosomal structures of frozen ram spermatozoa. *Australian Journal of Biological Sciences*, **28**, 153–9.

Whittingham, D.G. (1974). Embryo banks in the future of developmental genetics. *Genetics*, **78**, 395–402.

Wildt, D.E. (1992). Genetic resource banks for conserving wildlife species: justification, examples and becoming organized on a global basis. *Animal Reproduction Science*, **28**, 247–57.

Willoughby, C.E., Mazur, P., Peter, A.T. & Critser, J.K. (1996). Osmotic tolerance limits and properties of murine spermatozoa. *Biology of Reproduction*, **55**, 715–27.

Woelders, H. & Chaveiro, A. (2004). Theoretical prediction of "optimal" freezing programmes. *Cryobiology*, **49**, 258–71.

Woods, E.J., Liu, J., Derrow, C.W. *et al.* (2000). Osmometric and permeability characteristics of human placental/umbilical cord blood CD34+ cells and their application to cryopreservation. *Journal of Hematotherapy and Stem Cell Research*, **9**, 161–73.

Yokoyama, M., Akiba, H., Katsuki, M. & Nomura, T. (1990). Production of normal young following transfer of mouse embryos obtained by in vitro fertilization using cryopreserved spermatozoa. *Jikken Dobutsu*, **39**, 125–8.

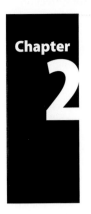

Chapter 2

Effects of antineoplastic and other medical treatments on sperm production

Marvin L. Meistrich

Introduction

When men who might want children are diagnosed with a serious disease that requires potentially sterilizing therapy, they need to have the proper information about sperm banking explained to them promptly after the diagnosis is made. This is particularly true of men with cancer, for whom the time interval between initial diagnosis and initiation of treatment is often just a few weeks or days. During this period, many tests are performed to determine the stage of disease, which dictates the treatment option. This period could well be used to bank sperm, but too often the issue of sperm banking is not raised until the treatment plan is finalized, presenting a dilemma: initiate treatment immediately or delay it until sperm can be banked. It cannot be overemphasized that, once the diagnosis is made and the probability that the patient will receive some form of sterilizing treatment can be estimated, a well-informed decision about sperm banking can be made at that time.

Some of the same drugs, in particular cyclophosphamide, used to treat cancers are also used in high doses in the treatment of nephrotic and autoimmune disorders. As a result, men with these diseases should also be given early information about the possibility of sperm banking. In the case of cancer, both the neoplastic disease and its treatment can interfere with normal reproductive function. Testicular cancer involves the gonad, and prostate cancer directly involves the reproductive tract. Even surgical treatment for these diseases results in damage or loss of these important reproductive organs. Retroperitoneal lymph node dissection for testicular and colon cancer, prostatectomy, and surgery involving the bladder neck may result in loss of the ability to ejaculate. Primary and metastatic tumors in the hypothalamus and pituitary can directly affect gonadotropin secretion, resulting in secondary hypogonadism.

Both chemotherapy and radiation cause toxic effects on the male gonads. If fertility is maintained or recovers, there remains the concern about the heritability of cancer and at least a theoretical risk of mutagenic alterations to germ cells caused by cytotoxic therapies. The loss of germ cells has secondary effects on the hypothalamic–pituitary–gonadal axis. Germinal aplasia reduces testis size and consequently testicular blood flow is reduced, so less testosterone enters the circulation (Wang et al., 1983). Since testosterone is a negative regulator of luteinizing hormone (LH) secretion by the pituitary, and LH is the primary stimulator of testosterone synthesis by the Leydig cells (Figure 2.1), LH increases to maintain serum testosterone levels. Thus after most cytotoxic therapies, with the exception

Sperm Banking: Theory and Practice, eds. Allan A. Pacey and Mathew J. Tomlinson.
Published by Cambridge University Press. © Cambridge University Press 2009.

of high-dose irradiation directly to the testis, serum testosterone levels remain in the normal or low–normal range and sexual function is rarely directly affected.

Normal spermatogenesis: kinetics

The testis consists of the seminiferous (or germinal) epithelium arranged in tubules and endocrine components (testosterone-producing Leydig cells) in the interstitial region between the tubules. The seminiferous tubules contain the germ cells, which consist of stem and differentiating spermatogonia, spermatocytes, spermatids, and sperm, and the Sertoli cells, which support and regulate germ cell differentiation (Figure 2.1).

Among the germ cells, the differentiating spermatogonia (some of the type A_{pale} and type B) proliferate most actively and can undergo apoptosis. Hence they are extremely susceptible to being killed by the cytotoxic agents. In contrast, the Leydig and Sertoli cells, which do not proliferate in adults, survive most cytotoxic therapies, although they might suffer functional damage. The later-stage germ cells (spermatocytes onward) are relatively resistant to killing. However, these cells are susceptible to mutagenic damage. The spermatogonial stem cells appear to be more resistant to killing by cytotoxic therapies than the differentiating spermatogonia but are more sensitive than the later-stage germ cells or the somatic cells.

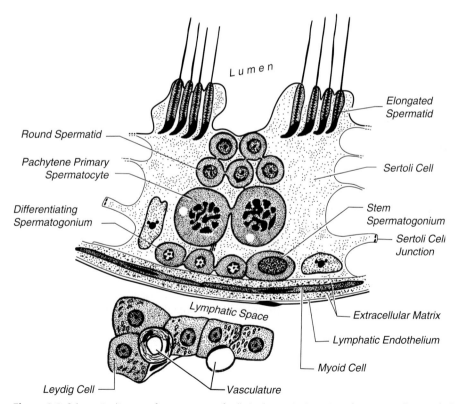

Figure 2.1 Schematic diagram of arrangement of cells in the testis. A portion of one seminiferous tubule and a cluster of interstitial cells are shown (Meistrich, 1986). Reprinted with permission from the *British Journal of Cancer*.

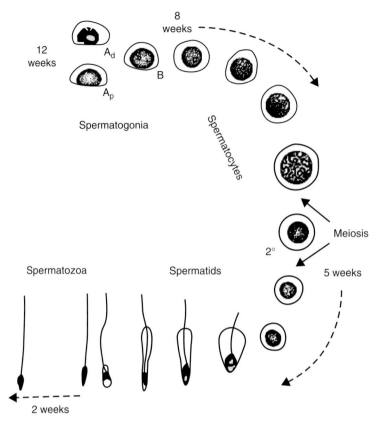

Figure 2.2 Sequence of spermatogenesis in the human showing the time it takes each cell type to become spermatozoa in the ejaculate. The type A_{dark} (A_d) spermatogonia are believed to be the reserve stem cells and the type A_{pale} (A_p) the active stem cells under normal circumstances. The type B spermatogonia, and possibly some of the A_{pale} cells, are the differentiating spermatogonia. The primary spermatocytes develop and undergo the first meiotic division to become secondary spermatocytes (2°), which rapidly undergo the second meiotic division to become spermatids. The spermatids undergo dramatic morphologic changes to assume the shape of spermatozoa before they leave the testis. Spermatozoa undergo a 12-day maturation period in the epididymis and vas deferens before they reach the ejaculate.

The relationship between the effects of cytotoxic agents on the testis and the consequences for the ejaculated spermatozoa is based on the kinetics of spermatogenesis (Figure 2.2). Once a stem cell becomes committed to differentiate, the kinetics of differentiation are precisely defined. Differentiating cells either progress along this time clock of differentiation or die. Thus for the first 12 days after the initiation of cytotoxic therapy, the sperm found in the ejaculate are derived from cells that were spermatozoa in the epididymis or vas deferens at the time of first exposure to therapy. Then during days 13–34, 35–58, and 59–85 the sperm produced were derived from cells that were, respectively, spermatids, spermatocytes, and differentiating spermatogonia at the time of initiation of therapy. After 85 days, sperm, if produced, must have been derived from cells that were stem cells at the initiation of therapy.

After cytotoxic treatment, sperm count diminishes with a time course that depends on the sensitivities of the different spermatogenic cells and their kinetics of maturation to sperm. The eventual recovery of sperm production depends on the survival of the spermatogonial stem cells and their ability to differentiate.

Table 2.1 *Testicular radiation doses from different radiation fields*

Radiation field	Disease	Testicular radiation dose (Gy)
Mantle	Hodgkin's	<0.05
Para-aortic lymph nodes	Seminoma, Hodgkin's	0.1–0.2
Hemi-pelvic	Seminoma	0.3–0.8
Pelvic	Hodgkin's	2[a]
Whole body	Leukemia (transplant preparation)	8–13[b]
Testis	Carcinoma *in situ* associated with nonseminomatous germ cell tumor in contralateral testis	20[c]

[a] Given as fractionated radiation over four weeks.
[b] Given as a single dose or in up to six fractions.
[c] Given in ten fractions.

Effects of radiation and chemotherapy on sperm production

Since the later-stage germ cells are relatively resistant to killing by cytotoxic therapies, and cells progress through spermatogenesis with constant kinetics, during the first two months of cytotoxic therapy, sperm counts may be only moderately reduced (Meistrich *et al.*, 1997). Between two and three months after the initiation of therapy, which is the time required for differentiating spermatogonia to become sperm, transient azoospermia appear even in patients not given highly gonadotoxic agents.

The testis receives irradiation when sites that are close to it are irradiated (Table 2.1). The dose to the testis is largely derived from internal scattering of radiation directed to nearby sites in the body and depends on the dose to the target field, the size of the target field, and the proximity of the field to the testis. Target fields not close to the testis, such as to the mantle, used in the treatment of early-stage Hodgkin's disease only above the diaphragm, result in only negligible radiation to the testis. Irradiation of the para-aortic lymph nodes results in doses of approximately 0.1–0.2 Gy. The hemi-pelvic and full pelvic fields deliver about 0.5 Gy or 2 Gy of scattered radiation to the testis (Hahn *et al.*, 1982; Jacobsen *et al.*, 1997; Dubey *et al.*, 2000). When pelvic irradiation is given, shielding of the testis is critical. High doses of radiation (>2 Gy) to the testis also occur in 30 percent of men receiving radiotherapy for soft tissue sarcomas in the thigh or hip area (Shapiro *et al.*, 1985). There are a few cancers in which the treatment includes the testis in the radiation field, resulting in very high doses of testicular radiation. These treatments include total body irradiation used in preparation for hematopoietic stem cell transplantation (Sanders *et al.*, 1996) and testicular irradiation for carcinoma *in situ* in the contralateral testis after orchiectomy for testicular cancer (Petersen *et al.*, 2002).

Whereas gonadal irradiation rapidly causes primary hypogonadism, cranial irradiation causes the gradual development of secondary hypogonadism over a period of years due to damage to the hypothalamus and/or the pituitary. This secondary hypogonadism can result from doses of 20 Gy or more directly to the pituitary, or a dose of 40 Gy or more to other parts of the head, which produces high levels of scattered radiation to the hypothalamus and pituitary. Sperm banking is advisable but may not be essential in these cases since hormone replacement therapy can compensate for reduced levels of gonadotropins.

The effects of different radiation doses on transient decreases in sperm count have been carefully evaluated after single doses of radiation (Clifton & Bremner, 1983) and following fractionated irradiation (Dubey et al., 2000), with similar results (Table 2.2). Doses to the testes above 0.15 Gy are required to produce any reduction in sperm count. Doses between 0.15 and 0.50 Gy cause oligospermia: the nadir of sperm count occurs 4–6 months after the end of treatment, and 10–18 months are required for complete recovery (Gordon et al., 1997). At doses of 0.6 Gy, azoospermia occurs, although sperm count usually returns to normal between 8 and 24 months after the end of therapy. Nevertheless, about 35 percent of men treated with radiotherapy for seminoma were not able to produce a pregnancy with their partners (Huyghe et al., 2004).

The benefit ratio (compared to cost or other factors) of sperm banking should be evaluated considering the short- and long-term risks of infertility and the possibility of genetic damage. Irradiation to fields not close to the testis carries very little risk of these outcomes, and so turning down the option of sperm banking is reasonable in these instances. Even irradiation to para-aortic fields carries little known risk. However, there are other considerations that the healthcare professional who is advising patients should mention. The tumor may not be responsive to that treatment or relapse might occur within a short time after therapy, before the restoration of normal sperm production and genetic integrity. Although the planned treatment may not have significant long-term effects on sperm production, the patient may have to undergo more highly sterilizing therapy (second-line therapy, high-dose chemotherapy, and hematopoietic stem cell transplant) before he has recovered sufficient sperm count and quality to bank later.

It is more difficult than was the case with radiation to determine the dose- and agent-specific response for the transient effects of different chemotherapy agents on sperm count reduction. Suffice to say that of the 24 cytotoxic agents that we have tested for reductions in sperm counts attributed to killing the differentiating spermatogonia in mice, only two did not have marked effects (Lu & Meistrich, 1979; Meistrich et al., 1982; da Cunha et al., 1985; Hacker-Klom et al., 1986; Bucci & Meistrich, 1987). Therefore, it is likely that almost all cytotoxic chemotherapy treatments, especially when they consist of combinations of several drugs, will have a transient deleterious effect on sperm count and quality.

Recovery of spermatogenesis after therapy

Frequently, following cytotoxic therapies, germ cells appear to be absent or nearly so (germinal aplasia); most of the tubules contain only Sertoli cells, and no sperm are found in the ejaculate. This induced azoospermia may be either temporary or prolonged, depending on the nature and dose of the cytotoxic agent. Chemotherapeutic agents differ markedly in their ability to produce prolonged azoospermia. Only the alkylating agents, and cisplatin, which acts similarly to alkylating agents in its ability to cross-link DNA, are capable of inducing long-term azoospermia as individual agents or as the main active agent in combinations. The specific chemotherapeutic agents and the doses of these agents that cause prolonged azoospermia are listed in Table 2.3.

If treatment is limited to the cytotoxic agents that do not cause prolonged azoospermia on their own (the first three groups in Table 2.3 and radiation), oligo- or azoospermia is transient, and normospermia is usually restored within three months after the cytotoxic therapy. However, if the more gonadotoxic agents are used, longer periods of azoospermia ensue. At lower doses of these agents, recovery to normospermic levels can occur within one to three years, but at higher doses, azoospermia may be more prolonged or even

Table 2.2 *Effect of different radiation doses on sperm count*

Testicular radiation dose (Gy)	Effect on sperm count
<0.15	None detectable
0.15–0.5	Transient oligospermia
0.6–2.0	Azoospermia (usually reversible)
>2.5[a]	Azoospermia (generally permanent)
8[b]	Permanent azoospermia in 85% of men

[a] Given as fractionated radiation over four weeks.
[b] Given as a single dose or in up to six fractions.

Table 2.3 *Antineoplastic agents that can cause or add to prolonged azoospermia in humans*[a]

Agents (cumulative dose for effect)	Effect
Chlorambucil (1.4 g/m^2) Cyclophosphamide (19 g/m^2) Procarbazine (4 g/m^2) Melphalan (140 mg/m^2) Cisplatin (500 mg/m^2)	Prolonged azoospermia
BCNU (1 g/m^2) CCNU (500 mg/m^2)	Azoospermia in adulthood after treatment prior to puberty
Busulfan (600 mg/m^2) Ifosfamide (42 g/m^2) Nitrogen mustard Actinomycin D	Likely to cause prolonged azoospermia, but always given with other highly sterilizing agents
Adriamycin (770 mg/m^2) Thiotepa (400 mg/m^2) Cytosine arabinoside (1 g/m^2) Vinblastine (50 mg/m^2)	Reported to be additive with above agents in causing prolonged azoospermia, but causes only temporary reductions in sperm count when not combined with above agents

[a] Modified from Meistrich *et al.* (2005). Note: The table in that reference incorrectly gave the dose of busulfan as 600 mg/kg.

permanent. Although the probability that spermatogenesis will recover decreases with the duration of azoospermia, a few men have recovered spermatogenesis after as long as 20 years of azoospermia (Marmor *et al.*, 1992). When the sperm count recovers after cytotoxic therapy, sperm motility appears to be normal (Pryzant *et al.*, 1993), and fertility is generally restored. However, if there is a long duration of azoospermia, the sperm count may sometimes plateau at less than one million per milliliter (Meistrich *et al.*, 1992).

The mechanism for the prolonged delay in recovery of sperm production is not known. The cytotoxic agents kill stem cells but studies in rats have shown that they can also damage the somatic environment of the testis, rendering it incapable of supporting differentiation of surviving stem cells (Zhang *et al.*, 2007). It has been proposed that the prolonged delay may be attributed to the requirement for the stem cells to first regenerate their numbers before initiating differentiation. Alternatively, the delay might be related to the repair of the somatic damage, as has been shown in rats, in which reversal of the somatic damage and restoration of spermatogonial differentiation can be achieved by transient suppression of testosterone (Shetty *et al.*, 2000).

Note that it is sometimes possible to choose, among nearly equally curative regimens, one that minimizes the doses of the agents (Table 2.3) that are most sterilizing. The use of ABVD (adriamycin, bleomycin, vinblastine, dacarbazine) instead of MOPP (nitrogen mustard, vincristine, procarbazine, prednisone) to treat Hodgkin's disease has dramatically reduced long-term gonadal toxicity (Viviani *et al.*, 1985) and is now the treatment of choice. The reduced risk of sterility has an effect on sperm banking decisions, but it is still possible that the tumor may be non-responsive or relapse may occur before sperm counts have returned to normal.

Genetic mutations in model systems and human spermatozoa

Many anticancer agents damage DNA, interfere with its replication and repair, or affect chromosome segregation in both rodent and human cells; all of these events could result in mutations. These anticancer agents have been shown to induce heritable mutations, including both single gene and chromosomal alterations, in germ cells of animals (Witt & Bishop, 1996). No induction of heritable mutations has conclusively been demonstrated in humans.

Based on the kinetics of spermatogenesis (Figure 2.2), mutations induced in post-stem cell stages of spermatogenesis will result in production of mutation-carrying sperm for only a few months. In contrast, mutations induced in stem spermatogonia will continue to produce mutation-carrying sperm for the lifetime of the male.

In male rodents, meiotic and post-meiotic germ cells are more sensitive to the induction and transmission of mutations than are stem spermatogonia (Meistrich, 1993). Therefore, mutational risks will be highest when a pregnancy occurs within one spermatogenic cycle (time for stem cell to become sperm) after the male is exposed to the damaging agent. The sensitivity of meiotic and post-meiotic cells to mutation induction is an important consideration in cases where a patient wants to start sperm banking after the initiation of chemotherapy. The agents that directly damage DNA, such as the alkylating agents, are expected to pose the greatest risk. Indeed, cyclophosphamide has been shown to induce genetic damage in spermatozoa in the epididymis that results in postimplantation embryonic lethality, although no gross malformations were observed in the surviving embryos (Qiu *et al.*, 1992). Meiotic cells are also at risk of induction of chromosomal abnormalities when certain anticancer agents, for example the topoisomerase II inhibitor etoposide, are used (Marchetti *et al.*, 2001). Stem cells appear to be less sensitive to mutation induction. Only radiation and several alkylating agents produce a significant frequency of single-gene mutations in mouse spermatogonia, whereas other tested chemotherapeutic drugs do not (Witt & Bishop, 1996). Radiation is the only agent that effectively induces stable reciprocal chromosomal translocations in stem spermatogonia (Meistrich *et al.*, 1990), which can be transmitted to offspring. Etoposide induces other chromosomal structural aberrations in stem spermatogonia. Although most of these aberrations will result in embryonic lethality, this still presents a theoretical risk to liveborn offspring (Marchetti *et al.*, 2006).

Because of the difficulty in assessing large numbers of offspring in epidemiological studies on humans, direct analysis of the genetic material of sperm has huge potential advantages for identifying probable heritable mutations in humans. Minisatellite-repeat-number mutations in human spermatozoa have been proposed as a useful marker for single-gene mutations. Indeed, minisatellite mutations were increased in offspring of men exposed to radiation from the Chernobyl accident (Dubrova *et al.*, 2002). However, the absence of increases in minisatellite mutations in spermatozoa (May *et al.*, 2000; Zheng *et al.*, 2000) or offspring (Rees *et al.*, 2006) of men after treatment with radiotherapy or chemotherapy indicates that the levels of such mutations are below the sensitivity of this technique.

Chromosomal abnormalities in human sperm can be measured by karyotyping after fusion of the sperm with hamster eggs or by fluorescence *in situ* hybridization (FISH). Structural chromosomal aberrations were present in sperm more than five years after the end of alkylating agent-based chemotherapy or radiation therapy, or both, indicating that they are induced in stem cells (Brandriff *et al.*, 1994). Numerical aberrations (aneuploidy) can show up to a fivefold increase during and shortly after (from <4 to <18 months, depending on the study) transiently sterilizing chemotherapy and then return to baseline (Martin *et al.*, 1999; Frias *et al.*, 2003). These results demonstrate that there may be significant genetic risks if conception or storage of sperm occurs during cytotoxic therapy, but that this risk declines after the end of such therapy.

Persistent DNA damage in spermatozoa

Numerous recent studies have utilized techniques that measure DNA or chromatin damage in sperm, including the COMET, sperm chromatin structure (SCSA), and the terminal deoxynucleotidyl transferase biotin-dUTP nick end labeling (TUNEL) assays (Morris, 2002). In general, these assays detect DNA strand breaks or damaged sites in the DNA that are susceptible to forming strand breaks under assay conditions.

The effects of radiation and chemicals that react with DNA on this type of DNA damage in sperm have mainly been studied in rodent models. The COMET assay has shown an increase in DNA strand breaks due to irradiation in sperm derived from all stages of mouse spermatogenic cells, reaching a maximum at the time that the spermatozoa would have been derived from irradiated differentiating spermatogonia (Haines *et al.*, 2002). Although lower levels of strand breaks were observed when the sperm were derived from stem cells, there was a persistent level of production of damaged sperm. In addition, the early-stage differentiating spermatogonia were shown to be sensitive to induction of damage by the SCSA assay (Sailer *et al.*, 1995). The SCSA assay showed that some alkylating agents can produce a high level of damage in sperm derived from cells that were post-meiotic cells at the time of treatment, but other alkylating agents produce persistent damage even in sperm derived from exposed stem cells (Evenson *et al.*, 1989, 1993).

Studies of DNA damage in human sperm following exposure to chemotherapy have been limited. Increased DNA damage in the sperm produced during treatment with fludarabine, a nucleoside analog, was observed by use of the COMET assay; however, at 11 months after completion of the therapy, there was no significant increase in DNA damage above the pretreatment level (Chatterjee *et al.*, 2000). One patient has been reported to have secondary infertility after treatment with cisplatin, etoposide, and bleomycin despite normal semen parameters but unusually high levels of DNA damage were shown by the SCSA assay (Deane *et al.*, 2004).

However, it should be noted that these techniques only measure what might be pre-mutational damage and most of the strand breaks could be repaired within the oocyte, so it is not known whether this damage in sperm carries a mutational risk to the offspring. It is also not known if these breaks, induced by cytotoxic treatment, have adverse reproductive consequences. However, in some studies, male partners of infertile couples had increased sperm DNA damage, which, in some cases, was correlated with poorer outcome of attempted pregnancies with in vitro fertilization (IVF) or intracytoplasmic sperm injection (Morris, 2002; Zini & Libman, 2006).

Effects on subsequent conceptions and offspring

Although rodent experiments and chromosomal analysis of human sperm by FISH show a higher risk of mutations when the sperm are derived from meiotic or postmeiotic cells than from stem spermatogonia, clinical reports of outcomes of pregnancies in which conception occurred while the father was undergoing cytotoxic therapy are too limited to evaluate the risks (Meistrich, 1993). Nevertheless, based on the rodent data and the aneuploidy in human sperm (Robbins *et al.*, 1997), there is likely a period of somewhat higher risk that extends from the start of cytotoxic therapy until at least 3 months after the last course. Because of the uncertainty in the data, patients should be advised to wait 6–12 months after the last course of therapy before attempting a conception or banking sperm, if they have not done so before treatment. After this time, the incidence of mutations is expected to be at the lower level found in sperm that were exposed to the mutagen as stem cells.

In humans, nearly all of the case reports, small series, and a few large retrospective case studies of the outcomes of pregnancies produced by survivors of cancer indicated no significant increase, above the background in the general population of about 4 percent, in birth defects or genetic disease in offspring conceived after cytotoxic treatment (Blatt, 1999). In most reports, conceptions occurred long after the end of treatment, and hence the sperm involved were derived from cells that had been exposed as stem cells. No increase in genetic disease was observed in 272 offspring from men who had been children or adolescents at the time of treatment and received alkylating agents or radiation proximal to the gonads (Hawkins, 1991; Meistrich & Byrne, 2002). In addition, 70 offspring from testicular cancer patients treated with radiotherapy and/or chemotherapy (most received cisplatin) revealed no apparent increase in congenital malformations (Senturia *et al.*, 1985). In a case–control study involving 41 000 children with congenital abnormalities, there was no higher incidence of paternal exposure to alkylating agents or radiation proximal to the gonads in the fathers of children with congenital abnormalities than in the fathers of the control group of children (Dodds *et al.*, 1993). The results from the atomic bomb survivor studies in Japan also showed no significant increase in genetic damage in more than 5000 offspring of men receiving significant radiation exposure (Schull *et al.*, 1981). These observations should reassure those who wish to have children following treatment chemotherapy or radiotherapy. However, in general, the power of these studies can only rule out a ≥twofold increase in abnormalities; the possibility of a small genetic risk that would increase genetic abnormalities less than twofold over background remains. Also, these long-term studies do not include many patients receiving the newer chemotherapeutic agents.

Still the most important reason for sperm banking is the risk of infertility after surgical or cytotoxic treatments for cancer and other diseases. At present there is no conclusive evidence for significant long-term genetic risks.

Acknowledgements

The author acknowledges Walter Pagel for editorial assistance and the Florence M. Thomas Professorship in Cancer Research for support.

References

Blatt, J. (1999). Pregnancy outcome in long-term survivors of childhood cancer. *Medical and Pediatric Oncology*, **33**, 29–33.

Brandriff, B.F., Meistrich, M.L., Gordon, L.A., Carrano, A.V. & Liang, J.C. (1994). Chromosomal damage in sperm of patients surviving Hodgkin's disease following MOPP therapy with and without radiotherapy. *Human Genetics*, **93**, 295–359.

Bucci, L.R. & Meistrich, M.L. (1987). Effects of busulfan on murine spermatogenesis: cytotoxicity, sterility, sperm abnormalities, and dominant lethal mutations. *Mutation Research*, **176**, 259–68.

Chatterjee, R., Haines, G.A., Perera, D.M., Goldstone, A. & Morris, I.D. (2000). Testicular and sperm DNA damage after treatment with fludarabine for chronic lymphocytic leukaemia. *Human Reproduction*, **15**, 762–6.

Clifton, D.K. & Bremner, W.J. (1983). The effect of testicular X-irradiation on spermatogenesis in man. A comparison with the mouse. *Journal of Andrology*, **4**, 387–92.

da Cunha, M.F., Meistrich, M.L. & Finch-Neimeyer, M.V. (1985). Effects of AMSA, an antineoplastic agent on spermatogenesis in the mouse. *Journal of Andrology*, **6**, 225–9.

Deane, L., Sharir, S., Jarvi, K. & Zini, A. (2004). High levels of sperm DNA denaturation as the sole semen abnormality in a patient after chemotherapy for testis cancer. *Journal of Andrology*, **25**, 23–4.

Dodds, L., Marrett, L.D., Tomkins, D.J., Green, B. & Sherman, G. (1993). Case-control study of congenital anomalies in children of cancer patients. *British Medical Journal*, **307**, 164–8.

Dubey, P., Wilson, G., Mathur, K.K. *et al.* (2000). Recovery of sperm production following radiation therapy for Hodgkin's disease after induction chemotherapy with mitoxantrone, vincristine, vinblastine and prednisone (NOVP). *International Journal of Radiation Oncology, Biology, Physics*, **46**, 609–17.

Dubrova, Y.E., Grant, G.R., Chumak, A.A., Stezhka, V.A. & Karakasian, A.N. (2002). Elevated minisatellite mutation rate in the post-Chernobyl families from Ukraine. *American Journal of Human Genetics*, **71**, 801–9.

Evenson, D.P., Baer, R.K. & Jost, L.K. (1989). Long-term effects of triethylenemelamine exposure on mouse testis cells and sperm chromatin structure assayed by flow cytometry. *Environmental and Molecular Mutagenesis*, **14**, 79–89.

Evenson, D.P., Jost, L.K. & Baer, R.K. (1993). Effects of methyl methanesulfonate on mouse sperm chromatin structure and testicular cell kinetics. *Environmental and Molecular Mutagenesis*, **21**, 144–53.

Frias, S., Van Hummelen, P., Meistrich, M.L. *et al.* (2003). NOVP chemotherapy for Hodgkin's disease transiently induces sperm aneuploidies associated with the major clinical aneuploidy syndromes involving chromosomes X, Y, and 18 and 21. *Cancer Research*, **63**, 44–51.

Gordon, W., Siegmund, K., Stanisic, T.H. *et al.* (1997). A study of reproductive function in patients with seminoma treated with radiotherapy and orchidectomy: (SWOG-8711). *International Journal of Radiation Oncology, Biology, Physics*, **38**, 83–94.

Hacker-Klom, U.B., Meistrich, M.L. & Gohde, W. (1986). Effect of doxorubicin and 4′-epidoxorubicin on mouse spermatogenesis. *Mutation Research*, **160**, 39–46.

Hahn, E.W., Feingold, S.M., Simpson, L. & Batata, M. (1982). Recovery from aspermia induced by low-dose radiation in seminoma patients. *Cancer*, **50**, 337–40.

Haines, G.A., Hendry, J.H., Daniel, C.P. & Morris, I.D. (2002). Germ cell and dose-dependent DNA damage measured by the Comet assay in murine spermatozoa after testicular X-irradiation. *Biology of Reproduction*, **67**, 854–61.

Hawkins, M.M. (1991). Is there evidence of a therapy-related increase in germ cell mutation among childhood cancer survivors? *Journal of the National Cancer Institute*, **83**, 1643–50.

Huyghe, E., Matsuda, T., Daudin, M. *et al.* (2004). Fertility after testicular cancer treatments: results of a large multicenter study. *Cancer*, **100**, 732–7.

Jacobsen, K.D., Olsen, D.R., Fossa, K. & Fossa, S. (1997). External beam abdominal radiotherapy in patients with seminoma stage I: field type, testicular dose, and spermatogenesis. *International Journal of Radiation Oncology, Biology, Physics*, **38**, 95–102.

Lu, C.C. & Meistrich, M.L. (1979). Cytotoxic effects of chemotherapeutic drugs on mouse testis cells. *Cancer Research*, **39**, 3575–82.

Marchetti, F., Bishop, J.B., Lowe, X. et al. (2001). Etoposide induces heritable chromosomal aberrations and aneuploidy during male meiosis in the mouse. *Proceedings of the National Academy of Sciences of the United States of America*, **98**, 3952–7.

Marchetti, F., Pearson, F.S., Bishop, J.B. & Wyrobek, A.J. (2006). Etoposide induces chromosomal abnormalities in mouse spermatocytes and stem cell spermatogonia. *Human Reproduction*, **21**, 888–95.

Marmor, D., Grob-Menendez, F., Duyck, F. & Delafontaine, D. (1992). Very late return of spermatogenesis after chlorambucil therapy: case reports. *Fertility and Sterility*, **58**, 845–6.

Martin, R.H., Ernst, S., Rademaker, A. et al. (1999). Analysis of sperm chromosome complements before, during, and after chemotherapy. *Cancer Genetics and Cytogenetics*, **108**, 133–6.

May, C.A., Tamaki, K., Neumann, R. et al. (2000). Minisatellite mutation frequency in human sperm following radiotherapy. *Mutation Research*, **453**, 67–75.

Meistrich, M.L. (1986). Relationship between spermatogonial stem cell survival and testis function after cytotoxic therapy. *British Journal of Cancer*, **53**, Suppl. 7, 89–101.

Meistrich, M.L. (1993). Potential genetic risks of using semen collected during chemotherapy. *Human Reproduction*, **8**, 8–10.

Meistrich, M.L. & Byrne, J. (2002). Genetic disease in offspring of long-term survivors of childhood and adolescent cancer treated with potentially mutagenic therapies. *American Journal of Human Genetics*, **70**, 1069–71.

Meistrich, M.L., Finch, M., da Cunha, M.F., Hacker, U. & Au, W.W. (1982). Damaging effects of fourteen chemotherapeutic drugs on mouse testis cells. *Cancer Research*, **42**, 122–31.

Meistrich, M.L., van Beek, M.E.A.B., Liang, J.C., Johnson, S.L. & Lu, J. (1990). Low levels of chromosomal mutations in germ cells derived from doxorubicin-treated stem spermatogonia in the mouse. *Cancer Research*, **50**, 370–4.

Meistrich, M.L., Wilson, G., Brown, B.W., da Cunha, M.F. & Lipshultz, L.I. (1992). Impact of cyclophosphamide on long-term reduction in sperm count in men treated with combination chemotherapy for Ewing's and soft tissue sarcomas. *Cancer*, **70**, 2703–12.

Meistrich, M.L., Wilson, G., Mathur, K. et al. (1997). Rapid recovery of spermatogenesis after mitoxantrone, vincristine, vinblastine, and prednisone chemotherapy for Hodgkin's disease. *Journal of Clinical Oncology*, **15**, 3488–95.

Morris, I.D. (2002). Sperm DNA damage and cancer treatment. *International Journal of Andrology*, **25**, 255–61.

Petersen, P.M., Giwercman, A., Daugaard, G. et al. (2002). Effect of graded testicular doses of radiotherapy in patients treated for carcinoma-in-situ in the testis. *Journal of Clinical Oncology*, **20**, 1537–43.

Pryzant, R.M., Meistrich, M.L., Wilson, E., Brown, B. & McLaughlin, P. (1993). Long-term reduction in sperm count after chemotherapy with and without radiation therapy for non-Hodgkin's lymphomas. *Journal of Clinical Oncology*, **11**, 239–47.

Qiu, J., Hales, B.F. & Robaire, B. (1992). Adverse effects of cyclophosphamide on progeny outcome can be mediated through post-testicular mechanisms in the rat. *Biology of Reproduction*, **46**, 926–31.

Rees, G.S., Trikic, M.Z., Winther, J.F. et al. (2006). A pilot study examining germline minisatellite mutations in the offspring of Danish childhood and adolescent cancer survivors treated with radiotherapy. *International Journal of Radiation Biology*, **82**, 153–60.

Robbins, W.A., Meistrich, M.L., Moore, D. et al. (1997). Chemotherapy induces transient sex chromosomal and autosomal aneuploidy in human sperm. *Nature Genetics*, **16**, 74–8.

Sailer, B.L., Jost, L.K., Erickson, K.R., Tajiran, M.A. & Evenson, D.P. (1995). Effects of X-irradiation on mouse testicular cells and sperm chromatin structure. *Environmental and Molecular Mutagenesis*, **25**, 23–30.

Sanders, J.E., Hawley, J., Levy, W. et al. (1996). Pregnancies following high-dose cyclophosphamide with or without high-dose busulfan or total-body irradiation and bone marrow transplantation. *Blood*, **87**, 3045–52.

Schull, W.J., Otake, M. & Neel, J.V. (1981). Genetic effects of the atomic bombs: a reappraisal. *Science*, **213**, 1220–7.

Senturia, Y.D., Peckham, C.S. & Peckham, M.J. (1985). Children fathered by men treated for testicular cancer. *Lancet*, **2**, 766–9.

Shapiro, E., Kinsella, T.J., Makuch, R.W. *et al.* (1985). Effects of fractionated irradiation on endocrine aspects of testicular function. *Journal of Clinical Oncology*, **3**, 1232–9.

Shetty, G., Wilson, G., Huhtaniemi, I. *et al.* (2000). Gonadotropin-releasing hormone analogs stimulate and testosterone inhibits the recovery of spermatogenesis in irradiated rats. *Endocrinology*, **141**, 1735–45.

Viviani, S., Santoro, A., Ragni, G. *et al.* (1985). Gonadal toxicity after combination chemotherapy for Hodgkin's disease. Comparative results of MOPP vs. ABVD. *European Journal of Cancer and Clinical Oncology*, **21**, 601–5.

Wang, J., Galil, K.A.A. & Setchell, B.P. (1983). Changes in testicular blood flow and testosterone production during aspermatogenesis after irradiation. *Journal of Endocrinology*, **98**, 35–46.

Witt, K.L. & Bishop, J.B. (1996). Mutagenicity of anticancer drugs in mammalian germ cells. *Mutation Research*, **355**, 209–34.

Zhang, Z., Shao, S. & Meistrich, M. (2007). The radiation-induced block in spermatogonial differentiation is due to damage to the somatic environment, not the germ cells. *Journal of Cellular Physiology*, **211**, 49–58.

Zheng, N., Monckton, D.G., Wilson, G. *et al.* (2000). Frequency of minisatellite repeat number changes at the MS205 locus in human sperm before and after cancer chemotherapy. *Environmental and Molecular Mutagenesis*, **36**, 134–45.

Zini, A. & Libman, J. (2006). Sperm DNA damage: clinical significance in the era of assisted reproduction. *Canadian Medical Association Journal*, **175**, 495–500.

3 Referring patients for sperm banking

Allan A. Pacey

Introduction

The interface between the sperm bank and the medical disciplines where men are first diagnosed with a medical condition, the treatment of which is a threat to subsequent fertility, is of crucial importance if sperm banking is to be managed successfully. During a workshop held by the British Andrology Society in 2002 (Tomlinson & Pacey, 2003), it was noted that the referral process often caused significant problems, with too little time to complete the banking process adequately or other complex problems presenting barriers to successful banking being achieved. Thus this chapter has been written with that in mind and in an attempt to discuss the process of referral and offer tips and suggestions as to how it might work more efficiently for patient benefit.

Who are the users?

Males are referred for sperm banking from a variety of different medical disciplines and after many different medical diagnoses where treatment with potentially gonadotoxic therapy is planned. To illustrate the point, Table 3.1 shows the breakdown of over 600 referrals for sperm banking in Sheffield from 1985 to 2006. This excludes sperm banking as part of planned assisted conception treatment and includes only those referred from other departments of nearby hospitals prior to another medical procedure where potentially gonadotoxic therapy was planned. Perhaps unsurprisingly, 79 percent of all referrals for sperm banking were following a cancer diagnosis and with testicular cancer and lymphoma accounting for 26 percent and 23 percent of the total, respectively. By comparison, there remains a steady trickle of referrals for men who require sperm banking as part of the management of other medical conditions, such as endocrine disorders (Silveria *et al.*, 2002), spinal cord injuries (Engin-Uml Stün, 2006), or the use of chemotherapy in the treatment of various dermatological conditions (Grunewald *et al.*, 2007). Sperm banking is also commonplace prior to vasectomy (Friedman & Broder, 1981) or at the time of vasectomy reversal (Practice Committee of the American Society for Reproductive Medicine, 2006), as well as before gender reassignment surgery (De Sutter, 2001).

The analysis of data from referrals to the sperm bank cannot, however, provide a complete picture of the number of men who would benefit from sperm banking. By definition it excludes those men where time pressures to start treatment precluded them from being referred, or those who were never identified as being at risk and therefore given the opportunity. There is some evidence that sperm banking may not be offered to all patients who would benefit from it. For example, Schover *et al.* (2002) sent a questionnaire to 718 oncology staff and physicians in the USA and found that, although 91 percent of

Sperm Banking: Theory and Practice, eds. Allan A. Pacey and Mathew J. Tomlinson.
Published by Cambridge University Press. © Cambridge University Press 2009.

Table 3.1 *Sources of referrals for sperm banking in Sheffield (1985–2006)*

	Percentage
Endocrine	1
Fertility-related	3
Gender reassignment	1
Multiple sclerosis	1
Oncology	
Bone marrow transplant	1
Brain tumor	2
Glioma	1
Leukemia	8
Lymphoma	23
Other hematology	1
Other oncology	7
Sarcoma	4
Testicular	26
Unknown	6
Other medical conditions	1
Pre-surgery (not oncology)	2
Renal	1
Rheumatology	2
Spinal injury	1
Unknown	1
Urology	1
Vasectomy	6
TOTAL	100

respondents agreed that sperm banking should be offered to all men at risk of infertility as a result of cancer treatment, less than 48 percent either bring up the topic or mention it to less than a quarter of eligible men. Similar data have been shown by Saito *et al.* (2005) in Japan, who found that, although many patients had been informed about the risk of infertility before cancer treatment, about half had banked sperm on their own initiative rather than following a specific instruction from their clinician. In Canada, Achille *et al.* (2006) interviewed both men ($n = 20$) and healthcare providers ($n = 18$) and found that problems in communication between doctors and patients could be a major deterrent to sperm banking. They found that men often lacked a clear understanding of their personal risk of infertility, and doctors did not work through with patients the importance of having children or potential benefits of banking sperm.

It therefore seems probable that sperm banks are underutilized and not all men who would benefit are getting access to them. One of the conclusions of Schover *et al.* (2002) was that "clearer practice standards could help oncologists increase their knowledge about sperm banking and avoid dependence on biased patient selection criteria." It is probable that this criticism could also be leveled at other medical disciplines where potentially gonadotoxic therapies are used, although there is currently no evidence to refute or confirm this.

Identifying men at risk of infertility

Clearly it is incumbent upon each clinical team that uses gonadotoxic agents to make sure that adequate processes are in place to identify at an early stage any men who might be at risk of infertility and where sperm banking may be appropriate. The key is that a referral should be as early as practically possible in the diagnostic pathway so that there is the maximum amount of time available for liaising with the sperm bank and arranging storage before therapy begins. Although this may seem inherently obvious, exactly when to initiate referral for sperm banking is an important strategic decision because, if it is made too late in the pathway, then the patient's treatment may have to be delayed in order to allow it to occur, and in the case of life-threatening conditions this may not be appropriate. Conversely, if the decision is made too early then patients may be being referred for sperm banking that ultimately may not be needed, with obvious consequences for already stretched healthcare budgets in addition to any unnecessary upset that the patient may experience as a result.

To assist in the development of local protocols, Figure 3.1 illustrates in broad terms a typical sperm banking process with timescales annotated on the key stages based on the experience of the two editors of this book. In summary, this suggests that the banking of up to three samples (see Chapter 6) could be achieved within five to seven days of the referral being received at the sperm bank. This assumes that the patient is ambulatory, that viral

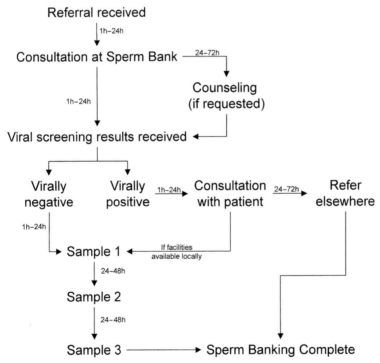

Figure 3.1 Flow diagram to show the process of sperm banking from the point of referral to all samples being cryopreserved. Timelines are meant as a guide only and will depend on the size and organization of services.

screening is negative (if performed), and sample production can be achieved without complication or surgical involvement, and that there are no issues of consent that leads the patient to request additional counseling in order to resolve them. Clearly the timescale may be shortened if fewer samples are stored or if viral screening (if required) is initiated prior to referral so that the results are available at, or shortly after, the time of referral. Conversely, the process can become more lengthy if additional counseling is requested by the patient, or if the patient is shown to be virally positive for human immunodeficiency virus (HIV), Hepatitis B or C, or human T-lymphotrophic virus (HTLV) (if performed) and the sperm bank does not have the facilities to process and store virally positive samples on-site (i.e. the patient needs to be referred elsewhere). Further delays may be encountered if the patient is unable to produce a sample by masturbation and more invasive surgical methods of sample retrieval are required (see Chapter 6).

Therefore in developing local protocols, it is a general guide that up to five to seven days should be factored into the time line in order to allow sperm banking to be completed adequately. In doing so, however, this may have adverse consequences for some patients who present with an acutely life-threatening condition that requires immediate treatment. Early dialog with the sperm bank should be able to establish whether or not it is possible to accommodate such requests as an emergency procedure should they arise, although clearly this situation is not ideal.

Guidelines for referral

Some sperm banks have facilitated the process of referral by developing specific guidelines in collaboration with the clinical teams that most commonly refer patients to them. These guidelines have the advantage that they can outline in advance the circumstances in which patients can be accepted (or rejected), as well as offer advice on anything that needs to be done before referral takes place. Clearly the details within such guidelines will be colored by the prevailing legal framework in which the sperm bank operates (country- or state-specific) as well as by local contracting arrangements or management issues. But with some thought it should be possible to develop guidelines that encompass most clinical scenarios.

Table 3.2 gives examples of guidelines based on the collective experience of the editors' own work in Sheffield and Nottingham in the UK. They cover, for example, the need for the sperm bank to have accurate information about the patient, his medical condition as well as advanced warning of any special needs or disability that need to be taken into account. For example, many sperm banks (Tomlinson & Pacey, 2003) have reported that a surprising number of patients have been referred who are impotent or unable to masturbate, perhaps owing to postsurgical pain or illness or because of moral, ethical, or cultural concerns. While such issues are not insurmountable – for example surgical sperm retrieval methods could be employed (see Chapter 6) – it could lead to avoidable delays if this was identified prior to referral for sperm banking since not all sperm banks have such facilities available as an emergency procedure.

Finally, it is important to recognize that guidelines for clinical teams are distinct from information sources specifically aimed at informing patients about the sperm banking process, although some information may obviously need to be duplicated between the two. Much of the information required by the sperm bank can be captured on a specific referral form, an example of which is shown in Figure 3.2.

Table 3.2 *Suggested topics for inclusion in referral guidelines for sperm banking*

General information
- Where the sperm bank is located and its opening hours
- The name and contact details of a designated person to contact
- Costs of sperm banking (e.g. any initial costs or annual costs)
- The mechanism of referral (e.g. referral form and where it can be obtained)
- Any legal (or contractual) restrictions on who can bank sperm
- Any legal (or contractual) restrictions on duration of storage

Information about the patient
- What information about the patient should be supplied (name, address, date of birth, diagnosis, etc.)
- The planned start date for any gonadotoxic therapy
- Whether the patient is ambulatory and can attend the sperm bank unaided or is an inpatient and requires assistance
- Whether or not the patient can provide the sample by masturbation or are more complex interventions required
- Details of any viral screening (if required)

Information about the referring clinical team or doctor
- Name and contact details of the referring individual
- Source of funding for the storage (initial costs and ongoing)
- To whom all subsequent correspondence should be sent

Information to be discussed with the patient in advance of referral
- The mechanism by which a sample for banking will be obtained (masturbation or more complex interventions)
- If the patient can masturbate the need for two to five days' sexual abstinence for optimum ejaculate quality (see Chapter 7)
- The need to sign legal forms at the sperm bank (if applicable)
- Any requirement to pay fees (if applicable)
- The need to make decisions about any consent to posthumous use of samples, embryo storage, or other aspects of storage and subsequent treatment

Patient information

The information about sperm banking given to patients may take many forms depending on their age, medical condition, or cognitive ability. Accurate information is an important part of the referral process so that males can make an informed choice about whether or not to bank sperm, what they can expect to happen during the process, and (if there is a choice available), which sperm bank to attend.

Sadly, there are few widely accepted templates of information sources available, although in the UK a working party of the Royal College of Physicians, Royal College of Radiologists and Royal College of Obstetricians and Gynaecologists (2008) has produced an information leaflet for men (and women) about the fertility preservation options prior to cancer treatment. This draws heavily on a booklet produced by Cancer Backup (Crawshaw *et al.*, 2005), which attempts to explain the issues surrounding fertility preservation and

Referral for Semen Storage

About the Patient	About the Referral

Surname:

First Name:

Address: (affix label if available)

Referring Consultant:

Date of Referral   /   /

Referred From (please tick one)

☐   Hospital 1
☐   Hospital 2
☐   Hospital 3
☐   Other

Date of Birth:

NHS No:

Hospital number:

Reason for Storage:

Diagnosis:

Date treatment starting: /   /

Has the patient been screened according to the "Guidelines for Referring Patients for Semen Storage"? y / n

If the results are available, please attach them.

If results are not yet available please inform us (below) of the date and time bloods were taken and where they were sent for analysis.

Declaration:
In my opinion the fertility of this man has been or is likely to become significantly impaired and I therefore recommend that his sperm be cryopreserved.

Signed:

Name & Address of patient's GP:

Address for Invoice:

Additional information (e.g. details about screening tests (see above) or any disabilities / special needs (including the need for translators)

For Sperm Bank Use Only
1st Appointment Details

Day	
Date	
Time	

Figure 3.2 An example referral form for sperm banking showing the key features of: full patient details; full details of the referring doctor; indication for storage and indication of urgency, including a medical opinion as to the likelihood of fertility impairment; information about funding (if required); and any special needs of the patient.

cancer treatment for younger adults. In a recent review of that booklet, Quinn (2007) noted that many doctors and nurses still lack the ability, and sometimes the courage, to adequately address the topic with their patients, highlighting both the need for information sources to be comprehensive and the need for staff to be appropriately trained.

In recognition of the fact that young people may find information booklets less accessible, much of the information contained within the Crawshaw *et al.* (2005) booklet is available online at www.click4tic.org.uk. Moreover, the Teenage Cancer Trust has recently produced a short DVD cartoon (see Figure 3.3) that may be viewed in preference to reading

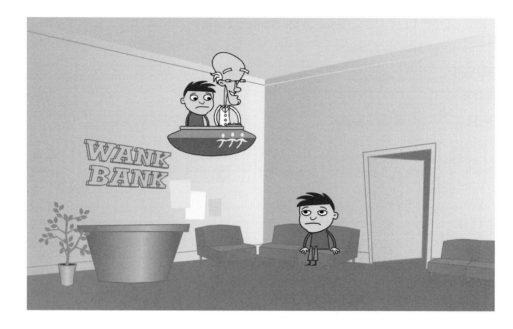

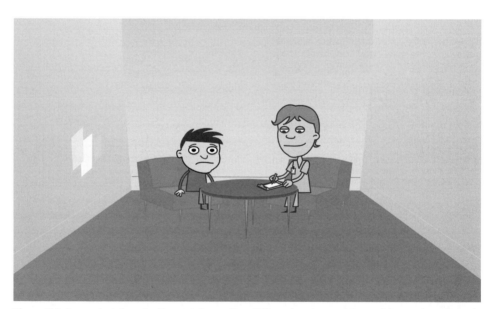

Figure 3.3 Screen shots from the Teenage Cancer Trust DVD produced to explain to adolescent boys about the process of sperm banking. The cartoon uses a comical doctor figure who explains the process including some of the more sensitive issues surrounding masturbation, consent, and later use of sperm in assisted conception treatments. While primarily intended for a UK audience, much of the subject matter is equally applicable to other parts of the world. Images reproduced with kind permission of Steve Donald (www.stevedonald.com) and with kind permission of the Teenage Cancer Trust (www.teenagecancertrust.org).

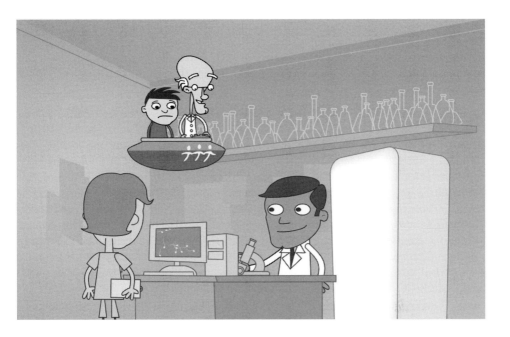

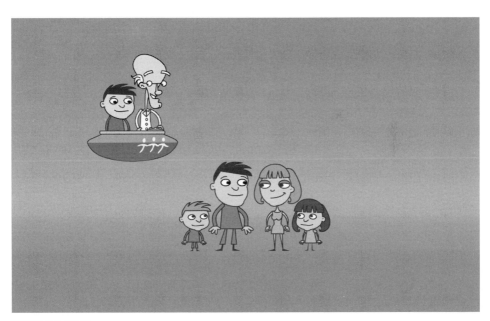

Figure 3.3 (cont.)

a leaflet. However, the effectiveness of such media, over and above a traditional written leaflet, has yet to be established.

Finally, the most appropriate time to give information about fertility and sperm banking has not been systematically examined. However, a study of young adolescents and their parents by Ginsberg *et al.* (2008) concluded that both want information to be given about sperm banking as early as possible. Interestingly, in this group, patients made their decision about sperm banking with the help of their parents 80 percent of the time. This may also highlight the need for information sources for the parents of young adults over and above that provided to the patients.

Problem areas

Although the process of referral for sperm banking is often straightforward, some cases will require special consideration. These include the referral of very ill (or unconscious) patients who are unable to attend the sperm bank in person, in addition to any problems that might be encountered in obtaining a sample from them. Many sperm banks may be understandably limited in being able to send staff to distant sites to see patients and collect specimens from them. Conversely, referring medical departments may not have adequate facilities for sample production or have sufficiently trained staff on hand to be able to take consent and adequately counsel the patient. Clearly, it would be advisable for such scenarios to be worked through in advance to ensure that adequate contingency plans can be put in place to deal with them. Such discussions could include the following.

- Who is responsible for taking consent and how is that information collected and communicated to the sperm bank?
- How the samples are to be transported to the sperm bank without compromising them (e.g. maintaining suitable temperature).
- What happens to specimens if the sample and the consent form(s) become separated? (e.g. it may be unlawful for a sperm bank to freeze a specimen without evidence of consent but not to do so may compromise the reproductive future of the individual and a potential lawsuit if the forms are later found but the sample was not frozen).

Clearly, very tight controls are needed to make sure the process works efficiently.

One problem area often highlighted is that of funding. In their review of facilitators and obstacles to sperm banking in Canada, Achille *et al.* (2006) identified that, for some males, the costs involved had been a major reason why they had not banked sperm (the cost of sperm banking is not covered by Medicare in Canada). Even in a state-funded healthcare system, such as in the UK, patients report surprise when they have to pay for their own sperm banking (Tomlinson & Pacey, 2003). This is not just in terms of the initial fee to store the sample, but the ongoing fee for maintenance of the sample in storage over the subsequent years. Clearly, any costs involved need to be discussed with the patient at the time of referral so that they are fully aware of them.

Other areas of concern are the need for sperm banks to remain in contact with men who have successfully banked for the duration of time that the samples are stored. Sperm banks often report frustrations (see Tomlinson & Pacey, 2003) that men with banked samples often do not respond to letters or change address in the years following successful banking. Often there can be a legal requirement for men to be contacted from time to time (e.g. in the UK current legislation requires sperm banks to conduct a biennial review of all material in storage and to check the nature and validity of consent). Given that men who are successfully treated for their disease will presumably attend follow-up appointments with the doctor who managed their treatment, it would seem logical at the point of initial referral to include some commitment between both medical teams (i.e. the referring clinician and the sperm bank) to undertake a joint approach to maintaining long-term contact with the patient. This is more than just to ensure that resources are used wisely and that banked sperm is not being kept unnecessarily, but also so that the patient has the opportunity to change and modify his consent over the course of his reproductive life if that is required and permissible.

Service evaluation

Service evaluation is an important aspect of modern healthcare, but published accounts of services evaluations in sperm banking services are not currently available. While some reports have published accounts of how many men who bank sperm subsequently return to use it (e.g. Kelleher *et al.*, 2001; Blackhall *et al.*, 2002; Agarwal *et al.*, 2004), such data offer a relatively blunt instrument by which to evaluate the success and customer satisfaction of the service. More informative are reports such as that of Saito *et al.* (2005), who showed that banking sperm had helped with the emotional battle against cancer. Clearly, better tools of service evaluation need to be developed to measure patient satisfaction so that different models of service delivery may be assessed.

References

Achille, M.A., Rosberger, Z., Robitaille, R. *et al.* (2006). Facilitators and obstacles to sperm banking in young men receiving gonado-toxic chemotherapy for cancer: the perspective of survivors and health care professionals. *Human Reproduction*, **12**, 3206–16.

Agarwal, A., Ranganathan, P., Kattal, N. *et al.* (2004). Fertility after cancer: a prospective review of assisted reproductive outcome with banked semen specimens. *Fertility and Sterility*, **81**, 342–8.

Blackhall, F.H., Atkinson, A.D., Maaya, M.B. *et al.* (2002). Semen cryopreservation, utilisation and reproductive outcome in men treated for Hodgkin's disease. *British Journal of Cancer*, **12**, 381–4.

Crawshaw, M., Glaser A., Hale, J. *et al.* (2005). *Relationships, Sex and Fertility for Young People Affected by Cancer*. London: Cancer-Backup.

De Sutter, P. (2001). Gender reassignment and assisted reproduction: present and future reproductive options for transsexual people. *Human Reproduction*, **16**, 612–14.

Engin-Uml Stün, Y., Korkmaz, C., Duru, N.K. & Baser, I. (2006). Comparison of three sperm retrieval techniques in spinal cord-injured men: pregnancy outcome. *Gynecological Endocrinology*, **22**, 252–5.

Friedman, S. & Broder, S. (1981). Homologous artificial insemination after long-term semen cryopreservation. *Fertility and Sterility*, **35**, 321–44.

Ginsberg, J.P., Ogle, S.K., Tuchman, L.K. *et al.* (2008). Sperm banking for adolescent and young adult cancer patients: sperm quality, patient, and parent perspectives. *Pediatrics Blood and Cancer*, **50**, 594–8.

Grunewald, S., Paasch, U. & Glander, H.J. (2007). Systemic dermatological treatment with relevance for male fertility. *Journal der Deutschen Dermatologischen Gesellschaft*, **5**, 15–21.

Kelleher, S., Wishart, S.M., Liu, P.Y. *et al.* (2001). Long-term outcomes of elective human sperm cryostorage. *Human Reproduction*, **16**, 2632–9.

Practice Committee of the American Society for Reproductive Medicine. (2006). Vasectomy reversal. *Fertility and Sterility*, **86**, S268–71.

Quinn, B. (2007). Book review *of Relationships, Sex and Fertility for Young People Affected by Cancer*. *Human Fertility* (Camb), **10**, 135–6.

Royal College of Physicians, Royal College of Radiologists and Royal College of Obstetricians and Gynaecologists. (2008). *The Effects of Cancer Treatment on Reproductive Functions: Guidance on Management. Report of a Working Party*. London: Royal College of Physicians.

Saito, K., Suzuki, K., Iwasaki, A., Yumura, Y. & Kubota, Y. (2005). Sperm cryopreservation before cancer chemotherapy helps in the emotional battle against cancer. *Cancer*, **104**, 521–4.

Schover, L.R., Brey, K., Lichtin, A., Lipshultz, L. I. & Jeha, S. (2002). Oncologists' attitudes and practices regarding banking sperm before cancer treatment. *Journal of Clinical Oncology*, **20**, 1890–7.

Silveira, L.F., MacColl, G.S. & Bouloux, P.M. (2002). Hypogonadotropic hypogonadism. *Seminars in Reproductive Medicine*, **20**, 327–38.

Tomlinson, M.J. & Pacey, A.A. (2003). Practical aspects of sperm banking for cancer patients. *Human Fertility* (Camb), **6**, 100–5.

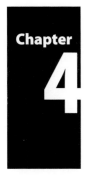

4

The psychological and psychosocial issues surrounding sperm banking

Marilyn A. Crawshaw

Introduction

Larger numbers of people diagnosed with conditions that threaten fertility or which require treatment with gonadotoxic therapies, or both, including in childhood, are surviving than ever before. However, outcomes do not necessarily include complete physical or cognitive recovery. The impact of potential or actual fertility impairment is an area that is increasingly pertinent for survivors. Knowledge about the longer-term consequences of fertility impairment as well as understanding of the impact of diagnosis and treatment need to inform practice from the start of contact with professionals. This chapter aims to aid that, concentrating primarily on the younger age group but drawing on research with adults from time to time.

The provision of sperm banking

The concerns of professionals involved in fertility preservation services from both oncology and reproductive medicine have been documented (Bahadur *et al.*, 2001; Coulson *et al.*, 2001; Wallace & Walker, 2001; Schover, 2002a; Cooke, 2003; Crawshaw *et al.*, 2004) and these fall into various themes, as follows.

- The challenges associated with communicating with, and relating to, people in shock following the diagnosis of a life-threatening illness.
- The effect of this on obtaining informed consent.
- The moral issues associated with offering a service for which there is no guaranteed success at a time when it is not required for current treatment.
- The lack of research into the impact of sperm banking at such a time, particularly when the patient is very ill.
- The difficulty of developing and maintaining relevant and up-to-date knowledge and skills where the incidence of referral is low.
- The particular difficulties attached to offering fertility preservation services to younger patients below the age of legal majority, including whether and how to involve parents or carers and partners.

Apart from barriers associated with time, cost, and facilities, there are some indications that clinician-initiated screening may take place on the grounds of medical factors (such as poor prognosis or aggressive illness) or social characteristics (gay men and those who are HIV positive) (Schover *et al.*, 2002a). In contrast, the limited research that has been undertaken so far with survivors of teenage cancer suggests that they have no such ambivalence and

Sperm Banking: Theory and Practice, eds. Allan A. Pacey and Mathew J. Tomlinson.
Published by Cambridge University Press. © Cambridge University Press 2009.

there is strong support for fertility preservation to be widely available (Schover *et al.*, 2002b; Crawshaw *et al.*, 2003). Marik (2004, p. 2680) brought home the personal costs of not having the chance to bank: "From time to time, a young man breaks into tears in my office when I tell him that he is azoospermic, that he missed the opportunity to preserve his reproductive capability, and that there is not much one can do after the sterilising surgery, chemotherapy or radiation was completed." Long-term follow-up studies with childhood and teenage cancer survivors suggest that concerns about fertility impairment increase as the threat to survival diminishes after the end of treatment (Blacklay, *et al.*, 1998; Schover *et al.*, 1999; Zebrack *et al.*, 2002, 2004), even where infertility was not medically predicted (Lozowoski, 1993).

The exclusion from sperm banking of those with a poor prognosis, for example, fails to take account of experiences such as those of John[1], whose opportunity to bank offered a source of hope when navigating treatment, a boost to resilience when coping with adverse thoughts and feelings, and a stake in the future even though, as it turned out, that stake was not likely to be realised:

John was only 14 when he was diagnosed with cancer but he'd always loved children and he wanted three – two boys and a girl in that order – when he got married. He had felt very embarrassed when his consultant asked him if he wanted to bank his sperm, especially with his mum and dad there, but he managed it OK. His treatment didn't go well. He had lots of infections and ended up having a lower limb amputation. His mum described the change in his personality from being happy-go-lucky to someone with mood swings that could include deep depression and outbursts of anger. At times, he was preoccupied with getting a girlfriend and worried about whether or not anyone would want him if he was infertile. When his deeper depressions lifted, he often talked about the way that he would explain his condition to a girlfriend and of how the "back-up" of the sperm in the bank would make him a more attractive partner than if there was none. As John moved into palliative care and toward his death, it is likely that he continued to draw on this hope.

The psychosocial impact of diagnosis

Diagnosis of a disease such as cancer profoundly changes a person's life and, often, the lives of those around them. It affects all spheres – the past, the present, and the future – and affects cognitive, emotional, and social function. Initial reactions are typically a mixture of panic, shock, despair, and uncertainty (Bennett, 2000; Ogden, 2001). As the new world of hospitals, specialists, medical terminology, medications, and treatments is entered "the daily activities and relationships that represent normality may temporarily disappear" (Bauld *et al.*, 1998, p. 121).

Although there is some evidence that young people in the wider population understand that cancer can be cured (Oakley *et al.*, 1995), it is nevertheless traumatic and often experienced as life-threatening to receive a cancer diagnosis. The person receiving the diagnosis, whether teenage or adult, will also be affected by the reactions of family members, partners, and others threatened by their potential loss. Adults, and especially parents, are perhaps most likely to see the spectre of death not cure. Parental adaptation is challenged by feelings of failure, punishment, and fear of death (Faulkner *et al.*, 1995; Langton, 2000; Grinyer, 2002).

Cancer is more than an illness. For many, it has cultural, religious, social, and psychological implications. There can be an accompanying sense of a battle going on within

---

[1] All the cases presented here include composite material from different research interviews; all the names used are fictitious.

between good and evil – evil being the cancer that needs to be fought off with the threat coming from within the body (part of you but alien) rather than outside (Zebrack, 2006). Feelings of loss of control of one's life and one's body are common.

By the time that patients arrive at the sperm bank, they will already have had to cope not only with the impact of the diagnosis but also the beginning of the cancer patient role. Whether inpatients or outpatients, most will already have been exposed to seeing other cancer patients, many of whom will have hair loss (typically a major concern of newly diagnosed patients) and be experiencing significant levels of physical illness or fatigue, or both (Edwards *et al.*, 2003). Even those who have prior experience of cancer patients describe the very different impact that it has when the viewer knows that they themselves are about to join those ranks. For many younger patients, this is their first introduction to serious illness and they vividly describe the fear that it engenders.

While the onslaught to one's sense of self and wellbeing at diagnosis can feel over-whelming, the immediate emotional task is simply to manage the impact sufficiently to take the next required step. The *et al.* (2000), through their work with adults, have described this process as starting with the existential crisis of diagnosis typified by a sense of despair and shifting toward a focus on therapy and the treatment calendar during the early stages of treatment. The visit(s) to the sperm bank can, of course, happen within hours, days, or (where banking takes place after surgery) weeks of diagnosis. Depending on the length of time since diagnosis, among other things, the shift into treatment mode may be well underway. However, it is important not to underestimate the potential for renewed crisis if information about the possible impact on fertility has not been relayed until well after diagnosis or separated from information about other treatment side effects, or both.

There is a small but growing interest in a gendered approach to understanding reactions to coping with health and disease, including cancer (Moynihan, 1998). While there are thought to be gender differences that relate to environmental experiences, biological pro-cesses, and treatment trajectories, it is perhaps the differences in coping styles that are most relevant to sperm banking. In a fascinating study that used the unusual method of analyzing men's and women's written narratives of being diagnosed with cancer, key differences for men were found, including that they: expressed themselves more matter-of-factly, less reflectively, and at less length than did women; were less likely to complain about not feeling "connected" to medical staff but more likely to report that their emotional needs had not been addressed; were more likely to underestimate their psychosocial needs and withhold or underreport symptoms; had more limited support networks, relying heavily on spouses (Salander & Hamberg, 2005).

These authors argue that gender differences may arise from earlier socialization and be reinforced and maintained by adult role expectations and obligations and "continuously constructed during interaction" (Salander & Hamberg, 2005, p. 685). Our identities are both social and personal but also highly gendered. These define and locate us as separate to, but part of, others. Although social identities derive from the cultures and communities of which we are a member, and are conferred on us by others, our personal identities represent our internalized version and "self concept." A cancer diagnosis invariably poses a deep-seated threat to both through the potential loss of "valued attributes, physical functions, social roles and personal pursuits … and their corresponding valued identities" (Charmaz, 1994, p. 269). For men who have limited experience of processing deeply felt emotions, this may come out in fear and rage as well as, or instead of, tears and sorrow. The former are more likely to generate hostility, disapproval, or misunderstanding in those around them and, paradoxically, increase the distance between them and potential caregivers.

Where male patients themselves (whether adults or aspiring adults) are immersed in masculine expectations of being strong, brave, and invulnerable, and/or such traits are expected by the professionals caring for them, the cancer diagnosis may pose a particular threat. The challenge for professionals is to be particularly vigilant at recognizing when they are themselves working from stereotypes rather than becoming attuned to the unique individual in front of them. Professionals may also need to be proactive in giving "permission" for men to express emotions and needs if they wish to, and to receive support while allowing those who wish to maintain their usual "masculinizing practices" to do so.

Coping with diagnosis

Research and practice experience together with personal testimony suggest that people can quickly start to move forward through unfolding reactions (Kubler-Ross, 1997) akin to people coping with grief (Parkes, 1996; Worden 2002; Parkes et al., 2003). As the reality of the diagnosis is increasingly understood, there will come a time of facing one's mortality (this is true for those around the patient as well) and coping with the fear and loneliness that are attached to that. Hope and optimism may start to return and defend against the (even if slightly) receding sense of fear unless the threat returns with failed treatments or relapse. Life patterns at all levels are affected and changes negotiated in the immediate, the medium, and the longer term. Although there may be movement backward and forward between the feelings generated, the overall progression to resolution is thought to be present. Evidence of moving beyond immediate impact can appear very quickly in some cases and thus it is important for sperm bank staff to be aware of this.

So-called "stage" theories have been developed to explain the process theoretically as it passes through an initial phase of shock, numbness, and disbelief to denial, avoidance, repression, or regression to anger (which may include anger displaced on to other people or events), search for some meaning to what is happening, and then finally to some form of resolution. The individual's unique pathway is thought to be affected by their level of cognitive ability, strength of self-concept and self-efficacy, level of access to reliable support systems (formal and informal), and overall socio-economic situation. Their experience is also likely to be mediated by their gender and culture. The younger the child or the more limited the cognitive function – say, for someone with learning difficulties or mental health problems – the more difficult it may be for them to comprehend the significance of the diagnosis at more than an emotional level. For someone who has prior low self-esteem and belief in their ability to affect or control the outcome of what happens to them, their reaction may be more inclined toward passive resignation or despairing hopelessness (Daniel & Wassell, 2002). For the isolated individual or the one whose adult life-role has entailed them giving support rather than receiving it, or in being "in control and strong" (for example, fathers or carers, or those who hold positions of responsibility at work), the lack of an ability to allow others to "hold" them emotionally and practically can make the cancer journey more difficult.

However, in reaction to concerns about the limitations of "stage" theories in explaining the fact that, for many people, emotional progress through their cancer journey does not appear to be linear, a "dual process" model of understanding has been developed (Stroebe et al., 2001). Within this model, individuals are seen to employ different but complementary reactions to their loss *from the start*. While being emotionally oriented to the situation and immersed in feelings (loss-oriented coping), Stroebe et al. (2001) suggest that people also employ "restoration-oriented coping" and that they oscillate between both states (men appear to be inclined to make disproportionately more use of restoration-oriented coping). Thus people may experience bouts of deep distress alongside working out ways to manage their treatment, sort out personal affairs, and start on the road to adjusting relationships. At an age-appropriate level, this may be manifest in the teenager who sorts out his favorite CDs to take into hospital in the midst of walking round in a daze and the adult who organizes his work diary while crying himself to sleep at night. It is important to the emotional health of anyone facing cancer to believe in future possibilities. Having what Charmaz (1994, p. 284) has called a "valued realm of action" available is an important way to preserve a valued self and, perhaps, to better allow the emergence of the needy self.

Decision-making and consent

It is in these early stages that sperm banking is typically offered. In cancer treatment, information has to be imparted straightaway about treatment regimens and side-effects as the need to enter treatment is usually acute. As cognitive function is diminished in response to the shock of the diagnosis, so is the ability to comprehend and process complex information. Recall of some facts may be very high (even where the person appears to be lacking in concentration or attentiveness at the time) but much more limited in others. The need to regularly paraphrase, summarize and revisit the facts, and not assume accurate or consistent recall, is therefore vital both over the immediate period and in the medium and longer terms. Decision-making is affected and may present at times more like compliance with actions suggested by those who have assumed some control through their professional expertise or their personal authority as parent, partner, or trusted friend.

Much mainstream literature implies that consent is a logical process in which patients weigh up harm, risk, and gain, and requires:

- Intellectual capacity to make and express a decision.
- Ability to acquire information and become informed.
- Ability to act voluntarily.
- Capacity to make, communicate, implement, and evaluate one's own decisions, understanding the risks and gains.

But medical facts about the cancer and its treatment, on top of the diagnosis itself, may in themselves induce shock or anxiety, reduce any calm and rational tendencies, and require confrontation of painful realities. The invoking of deep fears, hopes, and anguish mean that it is not unusual for ambivalence about decisions made in the immediate aftermath of a diagnosis to continue long after a decision has been made. In the immediate term, the potential for ambivalence can be lessened (though not removed entirely) and the more accurate absorption of facts can be facilitated when professionals take account of, and attend to, the patient's feelings about their situation. This includes the embarrassment of, or ambivalence about, masturbating in such circumstances.

Professional as well as patient anxiety may be raised at this time by the apparent shift in what is called the "locus of control" (Ogden, 2001; Kameny & Bearison, 2002). For teenagers and adults alike, the cancer diagnosis will shift their perceived sense of control dramatically away from personal self to the outside world whether that is to professional helpers, partners, or family members. Professionals may well feel more confident in influencing decision-making with regard to treatment regimens and entry into clinical trials – both of which require relatively complex processing of information by the patient – than in relation to sperm banking where the factual information to be processed is more straightforward but the evidence base about the emotional impact in the immediate and longer term of either banking or deciding not to bank is very limited. This will be compounded where the professional feels lacking in competence in relevant skills. One can see how it can be tempting to decide not to "trouble" John and others like him with the additional demands of sperm banking at such a time.

While it may not be possible or even appropriate to affect the shift in the locus of control around decision-making, any opportunities to restore control, no matter how slight, in other aspects of the process have therapeutic potential. This may include offering choice about:

- Who is present (professionals as well as family members or others) when the offer of fertility preservation is made.
- The point at which consent is taken.
- Who takes their consent, i.e. sperm bank staff or oncology staff or jointly.
- Where to produce the sample.
- Who to accompany them to the place where the sample is to be produced.

As Kameny and Bearison (2002, p. 169) have found, "staff can encourage their patients' feelings of mastery by giving them choices when possible."

Communicating the information

Deciding when and where to raise the topic of sperm banking and standards of communication at all stages of the process are key influences on outcome.

In our small-scale exploratory qualitative study of teenagers' experience of sperm banking conducted in two geographical areas in the north of England, there were differences among teenagers and among parents about how and when parents should be involved. Some favored parents being approached first, others favored teenagers and parents being told together, while others thought that parents should only be involved if the teenager agreed (Crawshaw et al., 2003). In the study by Schover et al. (2002a), 37 percent of professionals said that they would not talk to teenagers unless they had spoken to parents first, but the teenagers themselves wanted to be told on their own and then for their parents to be involved. This is understandable in the light of work such as that by Young et al. (2003), who found that professionals and parents preferred communicating with each other but the young people involved were sometimes then left feeling (unhelpfully) marginalized. Clearly, the younger the patient, the more likely it will be that parents will be invited to be present, but there are other models to consider and patient choice should be the deciding factor wherever possible.

Professionals are faced with a dilemma in that they rarely have much information about their patient or their family dynamics on which to decide how to raise this sensitive subject. However, the need for some prior family history-taking, even if only very brief, in order to avoid unhelpful assumptions is well illustrated by Andrew's story.

Andrew's parents had been separated for more than three years when Andrew's cancer was diagnosed. By 14, his relationship with his dad had deteriorated to the extent that he hated seeing him and couldn't understand why his mum thought it was so important that they kept in touch. He much preferred his step-dad with whom he got on well. He had grudgingly agreed that his dad could come along to the hospital when he was going for his test results. He had been feeling pretty rough for a few weeks but hoped that the doctor had sorted out what was wrong. He couldn't understand why his mum seemed so tense but thought it might be because his dad was with them. He soon found out once the doctor started talking about cancer. Everything went into a blur and all he could think of was that he was going to die – but not before his hair all fell out! Then the doctor asked his mum to leave the room and he was on his own with his dad and this doctor. He could hardly bring himself to tell his mum about it afterwards. The doctor had wanted him to masturbate into a pot and put the sperm into a sperm bank. His dad took off to the pub straightaway afterwards and told all that were there. Now everyone would know – all his mates, all the girls in his class. Andrew went to his bedroom saying that he refused to do it. When his dad called round drunk later on, his mum and dad had a blazing row. But once he'd gone, his mum sat with Andrew in the kitchen and started talking. She made it seem so much clearer. Andrew loved his new nephew, the way he gurgled and smiled – and he'd even had a go at changing his nappies, though he'd never tell his mates that! His mum explained that he might not be able to have children of his own because of the treatment that he was going to have, unless he put some sperm away in storage. He went the next day and managed it and got started on treatment.

In a large-scale study, involving 600 newly diagnosed adult cancer patients, Parle *et al.* (1996, cited in Bennett, 2000) found that unresolved concerns at this stage were a strong predictor of later anxiety and depression. This echoes earlier work in which adult oncology patients reported difficulties in eliciting the information that they wanted from medical consultations. Communication difficulties with members of the multidisciplinary team were heightened when there was lack of clarity about who had permission to tell patients what information.

The potential for communication difficulties, misinformation, and missed information-sharing is exacerbated further when staff from at least two distinct departments – in this case oncology and reproductive medicine – are involved in information-giving. The sperm bank staff need to know how the subject was raised and received in the oncology unit, what level of detail was imparted, and whether any difficult dynamics were encountered (including between partners or family members), and the oncology staff need to know how the process went at the sperm bank (with the patient's permission).

There is of course also the question of professional gender. Does it matter whether or not the professional helper is male? The evidence is inconclusive. While it appears to be the case that female patients generally prefer a female doctor, it is much less clear in relation to males. The findings from one study suggested that shared gender was of less importance than non-gender related attributes of respect, warmth, openness in information sharing, friendliness, and humor (Crawshaw *et al.*, 2003).

The importance of speaking clearly, without jargon, and directly to the person involved rather than to those accompanying him (regardless of the age of the patient or whether English is their first language) is well researched (Fallowfield *et al.*, 1995; Culley *et al.*, 2004). Striking the balance between being friendly and relaxed, but not overfamiliar, is an important additional skill.

Bennett's (2000) excellent summary of work in this area, together with other work, highlights the following attributes for enhancing communication, information exchange, and higher recall both at the time and in its aftermath.

- Using open rather than closed questions.
- Offering nonverbal cues indicating willingness to share information and discuss issues.
- Paying attention to the way that the content of verbal exchanges is framed.
- Using simple, clear, jargon-free language.
- Encouraging people to ask questions.
- Being alert to potential bias arising from cultural or gender stereotyping.
- Giving the most important information at the beginning and end of consultations.

- Regularly paraphrasing and summarizing in order to check understanding.
- Offering emotional support alongside the imparting of potentially distressing or disturbing information.

There is evidence to suggest that young people and adults prefer to receive information than to have it withheld, even when the information is painful to hear. Receiving information also appears to reduce uncertainty and help people to understand their situation better (Neville, 1998). The stuty by Schover *et al.* (2002b) of 14–40-year-olds found that those who discussed cancer-related infertility with a health professional had greater knowledge about it *and* were more likely to bank their sperm.

There may sometimes be a temptation on the part of professionals to withhold some information, fearing overload of their patients or fearing that the limit of their capacity to hear bad news has been reached. It is doubtful that anyone being told of cancer side effects or risks associated with sperm banking will find them easy to hear about: that is not the same as not wanting to know. Similarly, although additional information will need to be imparted over time that does not mean that preliminary information should be withheld.

Why do teenagers and men choose to bank their sperm?

Little is known about why teenage and adult males opt to bank sperm at a time when we might expect that their focus is on survival. It is not known how widespread the knowledge is in the wider population that infertility may be a side effect of cancer and its treatment, but it is likely that many receiving a cancer diagnosis are hearing for the first time that their fertility may be affected.

In a small qualitative study, explanations for the motivation to bank were located, not surprisingly, in the desire to preserve reproductive choice for adult life (Crawshaw *et al.*, 2003). All the participants had thought about being a father prior to becoming ill albeit in differing amounts of detail. In the study by Schover *et al.* (1999) of 132 adults, a majority of the survivors were interested in having children, especially if they were childless at the time of diagnosis. Grinyer (2002, p. 61) also describes the impact for some men right from the beginning of hearing that there may be permanent fertility impairment: "Fertility was for George a bigger issue in the weeks after diagnosis than the cancer diagnosis. He minded more the prospect of not being able to have children than he minded having the cancer diagnosis because I think he believed that he would survive the cancer diagnosis but he knew that he would almost certainly be rendered infertile through therapy." Sadly, George did not survive but he had been able to bank his sperm.

This reflects research that has been conducted elsewhere about children and young people's life ambitions (Fraser *et al.*, 2006) and about the strongly pro-natalist culture in some communities (Culley *et al.*, 2004). Although it is tempting to think that it is primarily girls who daydream about parenthood, it is perhaps the expectation about *what* is involved in parenting that differs between the sexes more than the desire to become a parent in itself.

However, Green *et al.* (2003) have pointed out that the news that fertility may be impaired (whether at diagnosis or at a later stage) often comes at a time when many people are not actively considering fatherhood. The intensity of the expectation and desire to become a father (or, indeed, to become a father again) may affect the intensity of the threat experienced when that possibility is challenged. This in turn may explain why some decide against sperm banking. The decision may also be affected by the level and type of cancer-related symptoms that are being experienced while others may simply passively comply with the suggested action as part of their perceived "routine" preparation for treatment. Some, like Hanif, will be more actively influenced by significant family members or professional advisors.

Hanif went from being a fit and healthy 16-year-old to being confined to his bed within a matter of days. The only way he could tolerate the level of pain in his head was by lying prone. By the time he was offered the chance to bank sperm within hours of his cancer diagnosis, he couldn't really take it in. On top of everything else, he was now being asked to travel across the city to another hospital where he would have to masturbate. His initial response was to say "No," but his consultant asked him to think about it and said she'd call back in an hour or so. He lay and thought about what she'd said. It had been good hearing her talk about what he wanted when he was an adult – it meant she thought he might live, after all. He liked the way that she spoke to him quietly and gently on his own with the curtains drawn round for privacy. She made it clear that it was his decision at the end of the day. When his dad came in, he reminded him of all those times that he'd talked about being a dad some day, playing football and teaching his children how to swim like his dad had done with him. He decided to give it a go. He travelled in his dad's car, lay down in the back seat, and he had to lie on his side on the couch in the examination room – but he managed it. Now, two years later, Hanif is in remission. He still doesn't know whether he is fertile or not – he prefers not to find out just yet – but he derives a lot of comfort from knowing that he has fertile samples in the sperm bank.

The greater that the impact of the cancer diagnosis has on the individual, and the younger they are, the greater the potential significance of "others" who may be in a better position either cognitively or emotionally to be able to hold on to the longer-term significance of the choice being offered. The importance of not taking the person's first decision as final is clear.

However, the decision to bank may not be wholly related to a desire to retain reproductive choice. Pacey, a cancer survivor as well as a scientist working in the field of assisted conception, has written about his own motivation to bank for "non-reproductive" reasons:

Looking back, I can only now explain my decision to bank sperm as something positive to do at an otherwise emotionally negative time.   (Pacey, 2003, p. 327).

This accords with what Neville (2000) has called the "promotion of hopefulness," the degree to which we possess the comforting and life-sustaining belief that we have a future.

Pacey (2003, p. 1354) cites fellow survivors whose motivations he also categorized as non-reproductive, including the man whose reason was to "wipe the smile off his oncologist's face," the gay man who did not want to disclose his sexuality, and another who wanted to preserve his masculinity. He went on to speculate that "maybe simply knowing that their sperm is somewhere safe, irrespective of what decisions they may or may not make about fathering, is a psychological benefit to men" (Pacey, 2003, p. 1354), it may be rational (investment against risk) but may also be "to avoid regretting it later;" it may be passive (because the doctor told me to do it) or it may represent the chance to wrest back some of the shifted "locus of control" by squeezing some personal control out of a situation where control has gone (Pacey, 2003, p. 1354).

How do people cope?

Coping with potential infertility as well as cancer involves an ongoing appraisal of the degree of threat that it poses at any one time to the impact on the individual's self-concept, life aspirations, and life opportunities. As such it is a personal construct within a specific context.

When a threat is experienced, our defense mechanisms seek to repel it in order to survive, and coping strategies kick into play. The psychological task for the individual is to reduce the perceived threat and that is typically done by altering our personal relationship to it.

Various models for understanding *how* people cope with life-threatening illness have been developed, which put the flesh on *why* people cope in the way they do. Bauld *et al.* (1998) outline three types of coping that might be of help in understanding possible reactions at this time:

- "Non-productive and denial or avoidance" (sometimes called "emotion-focussed") strategies, including worrying, wishful thinking, ignoring the problem, self-blame, and keeping to oneself.
- "Problem-focussed" strategies, including active information-seeking, focussing on the positive, seeking physical recreation, and being socially connected.
- "Coping by reference to others" strategies, including seeking help from peers, professionals, and others, spiritual support.

The greater the level of threat that is experienced the more intense the use of coping strategies will need to be. Those using the first type listed above are employing emotions to reduce the threat by changing the way that they *feel* about the threat – either expressing their feelings (e.g. crying, being angry) or suppressing them (being aloof, acting as if nothing is happening) or actively seeking emotional comfort (from people or from aids such as alcohol). Those using the second type listed are seeking to reduce the threat by changing the threat itself – either by defusing it (e.g. increasing other activity as an antidote) or by actively confronting it (seeking information about it, starting complementary interventions), and so on. We might expect that the former would be more indicative of the "loss-oriented" phases of the Stroebe *et al.* (2001) dual process theoretical understanding and the latter of "restoration-oriented" phases (see earlier). Given men's apparent tendency to use more problem-focussed coping strategies, this may go some way to explain the research of Moynihan *et al.* (1998) with men with testicular cancer which found that, on the whole, they neither wanted counseling around the time of diagnosis nor benefited from it if they accepted it.

Clearly, within this explanation, the third type of coping strategy listed earlier could be used contemporaneously with either of the first two as well as being a stand-alone strategy. While our existing coping approaches are suspended in the immediate aftermath of receiving a diagnosis and prior to new strategies being formulated, the reliance on the third type of coping stratregy will typically be greater to reflect the dramatic shift of the "locus of control" (see earlier). This also accords with the findings of Neville (1998), with teenagers with cancer, of the importance of *perceived* social support as a stress buffer and a predictor of reduced levels of uncertainty and associated psychological distress.

There is active debate about how far coping styles are related to personality traits (i.e. displaying familiar traits to a much greater degree of intensity than usual) or whether they are a reaction to the state (situation) that the individual is confronted with (and therefore traits may be displayed which are less typical for that individual) (Miller *et al.*, 1996).

How should professionals respond to different coping styles?

Some suggest that it is appropriate at times for professionals and carers to challenge individuals' coping strategies – especially those which are seen as unhelpful, such as denial, avoidance, and repression. Indeed, the use of the term "nonproductive" by Bauld *et al.* (1998) itself carries negative connotations and implies that a different approach would be "better." Neville (2000), in her research with teenagers with cancer, turned this on its head by suggesting that what she more positively frames as "adaptive denial" may actually serve a protective function by employing a positive, optimistic outlook on life instead of concentrating on illness. Green *et al.* (2003) reported that none of the adults (aged 19–32) in their study could recall a health professional challenging their style of coping (and different styles were employed by different participants) and they experienced this positively – that the professionals were respectful of them and allowed them to find their own way through. When this works, it could indeed be constructive and suggests a person-centered approach rather than an expert-led model. It might therefore be timely for "nonproductive and denial or avoidance" strategies to undergo a rebranding that recognizes their importance in the arsenal of strategies that people draw on.

On the other hand, there is growing though small-scale evidence to suggest that people may deal differently with matters associated with sexual activity and fertility than other aspects of their posttreatment health and wellbeing. Teenagers have difficulty raising issues of sexual function or reproductive health difficulties with their doctors (Malus *et al.*, 1987). Adults, too, find it difficult to raise such matters with professionals (for a brief review see Grinyer, 2002, pp. 73–5) and professionals themselves appear to find it a particularly difficult area to manage (Heiney, 1989; Senanayake *et al.*, 2001; Stead *et al.*, 2001). It is possible that some patients at least would like the subject raising proactively with them by professionals, and at an earlier stage than that at which they may actively contemplate parenthood – after all, impaired fertility may affect sexual identity, sexual activity, and life planning, not simply fertile identity.

Adam had many questions that he wanted answers to about sex and about his fertility once the treatment had finished. One time, he remembered joking with his social worker about how he'd be able to go "behind the bike sheds" with girls without having to worry now. He'd hoped that she'd realize that he wanted to talk about it but she laughed and just asked him how many girlfriends he had anyway. And when he went for follow-up appointments, his consultant always asked him if there anything else that he'd like to talk about but he didn't dare take the risk of bringing this up in case he didn't mean that he could ask her about sex.

Professional intervention at diagnosis and sperm banking needs to be cognisant of these matters if it is to help teenagers and adults alike to move more readily from acute discomfort into commitment to treatment and adaptation to symptoms. Professionals should seek to understand, acknowledge, and help maximize the individual's coping strategies rather than to interrupt or alter them – that is, work to reduce anxiety and threat levels rather than raise them.

The experience of sperm banking

Very little research has been conducted into the *experience* of being offered fertility preservation at or around a diagnosis of cancer or other conditions requiring cytotoxic therapy and of sperm banking itself. However, information-sharing about a range of facts associated with fertility preservation may ease stress, reduce uncertainty, and lower anxiety at the time of banking, providing they are clearly expressed and that the quantity is not excessive. This might include verbal and written information about the following.

- The quality of the sample.
- How many samples are banked and where.
- How many treatments the samples might support.
- The frequency with which future contact will be offered (including semen analysis).
- Whether or not any storage costs will be incurred.

How and when to give such information, and who should give it, is of course difficult to determine. The provision of supplementary written information is increasingly advocated and studies have shown that patient recall is better after receiving written as well as verbal information than if verbal information alone is given (for a review, see Arthur, 1995). This may be particularly pertinent given work such as that by Beaver and Luker (1997), which found that the initial shock of a cancer diagnosis may, for some, limit recall and retention of verbal information. However, it has been suggested that the majority of information leaflets currently in use in health settings are too difficult to comprehend, especially given the low levels of literacy in the wider population. It is crucial therefore that information is tested for "readability" using the various schemes now available. Similarly, the use of web-based information-sharing is increasingly rapidly and there are a number of new initiatives aimed at teenagers and/or adults (for example www.click4tic.org.uk; www.fertilehope.org; www.planetcancer.org; www.laf.org; www.ulmanfund.org). They too will need to be alert to "readability."

Attention to detail in information giving is also pertinent if experiences such as those of Jamie are to be avoided.

Jamie went with his mum and auntie to the sperm bank. Although the staff were expecting him and were very friendly, nobody seemed to know what to do with his mum and auntie. In the end, they came through with him when he saw the nurse to fill out the consent form. All still felt distressed more than 18 months later by the memory of when she asked Jamie what he wanted them to do with his sample if he died. He felt that it confirmed his worst fears. She didn't explain that everyone was asked that question and it wasn't because he had cancer. And then no one told him that there was a choice of specimen pots available. He was right-handed but the cancer was in his right arm. By the time he'd struggled to produce a sample, he was so agitated that he then knocked it over and had to start all over again. When he'd finished the second time, he realized that no one had told him what happened next. After waiting a while, he decided to go and find somebody. A doctor he'd never seen before told him to leave it in the room. He's been worried ever since about whether or not it really was his sample that they put in the freezer. It was more than a year later before Jamie talked about his experience with anyone. A favorite uncle had to give a semen sample as he and his wife were having difficulty conceiving. When he came round to Jamie's house on his way back from the hospital, he was telling Jamie's mum and dad all about it. Jamie got him on his own later and plucked up the courage to tell him about his own experiences – it was such a relief.

It takes little imagination to be alert to the embarrassment and ambivalence among men as well as teenagers at having to masturbate in these circumstances. It is crucial also to be alert to the possibility of experiencing it as "shameful" as that contains the potential for longer-term harm. Masturbation is associated with sexual activity but is also overlain with disapproval by some religions and some parenting approaches (Ryan, 2000). It is, of course, generally an even more private act than sexual intercourse and typically done without anyone else's knowledge at the time. This needs to be acknowledged by sperm banking services in as much as the room and surroundings should be as respectful to the act as possible.

Jacob's experience compounded his feeling that he was doing something shameful.

Jacob couldn't shake off the feeling that he was doing something quite bizarre and rather seedy by going to the sperm bank the day after being told that he had cancer. It was made infinitely worse when he was shown into a room which was clearly used as an office at other times. There was a paper sheet over an armchair and he blushed when he realized why it was there – not that he could imagine masturbating while sitting on an armchair anyway. Although he could lock the door, he could still hear people moving around outside and could even hear their conversations. He noticed a hardbound copy of a girlie magazine and was sickened to see how well-thumbed and grubby it was. He couldn't wait to get out of there and have a hot shower.

When we are diagnosed with an illness that strikes fear in the way that cancer does, we are already coping with being in a situation that none would envy. When that is overlain by the possibility that infertility will also result, we are also coping with acquiring a doubly stigmatized identity. It is likely that the impact of fertility impairment acquired through medical treatment will differ in some ways to the impact on people finding out as adults that they are unlikely or unable to conceive for some other reason, so there may be limited transferable material from which to draw. Nevertheless, male infertility is thought to be experienced by many men as striking at their sense of manhood, their virility, and hence their sense of potency (Mason, 1993; Monach, 1993; Lee, 1996). For young men moving toward adulthood in particular, their identity is likely to be increasingly bound up with this aspect and preoccupation with sexual prowess has been documented (Coleman & Hendry, 1999).

Do they regret their decision?

Broome and Allegretti (2001) reported on spontaneous discussion with two young men taking part in their study on entry into clinical trials for people undergoing bone marrow transplants. Both regretted their decision not to bank. In our small qualitative study, two of the young men had decided against trying to bank and one was already regretting his decision less than two years later. Another who had wanted to bank but could not get erections (and no alternative retrieval method was offered) remained sad about his failure to produce a sample.

But the impact of fertility does not end with the provision of a sperm banking service. Just as one's relationship to the decision about whether or not to store may continue to emerge and develop, so too might the significance of the banked sperm and the impact of the possible fertility impairment and any associated sexual and relationship difficulties. This unfolding understanding will be unique to the individual, but it is for the professionals to recognize that it may prove complex and may result in a need for medical, scientific, and psycho-social services over the coming months and years (Schover, 1997; Cooke, 2003).

The unfolding experience

Looking at the research from long-term survivor studies may also shed some light on an understanding of how best to provide services at the start of the cancer journey, regardless of whether or not the cancer is eventually survived.

With teenagers, the challenges of adolescence and associated life transitions run alongside the challenges of cancer. The transition to adulthood is marked by key shifts in relationships within the family and with peers, increased emotional and social independence, changing education and work-related experiences, changes in financial situation, a developing approach to morality, and a growing awareness of sexual identity (Coleman & Hendry, 1999).

For the adult whose life situation and attainment of roles may be less fluid, there are also life challenges and transitions to negotiate.

For both groups, the "tasks" can include:

- Returning to school or work.
- Actively picking up earlier social or family roles where appropriate.
- Re-establishing peer relationships.
- Integrating new peer relationships (e.g. with other survivors) into ongoing life.

- Managing new or existing romantic relationships in the light of the general cancer experience and the specific experience of impact on fertility and/or sexuality.
- Establishing healthcare patterns, including follow-up appointments.

All carry potential for new understandings as well as potential for crisis or threat – and require active ongoing appraisal of the meaning of cancer and fertility to the individual in each unfolding situation. As the threat to life recedes, other threats may takes its place, such as those posed by scars, amputations, loss of friends, fertility, insurance difficulties, education or employment difficulties, and other people in one's circle being diagnosed with cancer.

Generally speaking, the research suggests that teenage cancer survivors cope well with their experience (Eiser 1998; Self, 2006), though this is a lively area of debate. Some have suggested that there is a significant minority who fare badly (for useful reviews see Kameny & Bearison, 2002; Zebrack et al., 2002).

Zebrack (2006, p. 223) has concluded that "Positive psycho-social adjustment is associated with an ability to integrate the experience into one's self concept by deriving meaning from the cancer experience, creating changes in life priorities or accepting one's mortality." Blacklay et al. (1998) suggest that regular checks offer the opportunity to monitor physical and emotional wellbeing, to offer additional information, and to influence health behavior by encouraging health-promoting activities and discouraging health-compromising behaviours: "understanding the possible effects of chemotherapy on fertility may allow survivors to come to terms with their situation and limit the risk of emotional disappointment" (Blacklay et al., 1998, p. 341).

However, there may also be some differences in coping patterns that are unique to fertility (Lozowoski, 1993; Roberts et al., 1998; Green et al., 2003) and which may go some way to explaining survivors' apparent reluctance to actively seek information about their fertility status through semen analysis. There is also more work to be done before the impact on what Puukko et al. (1997) call one's "inner sexuality" is understood, including how far this might explain the apparent lower than average incidence of teenage and childhood survivors who go on to establish long-term adult relationships and have children.

Neville (2000) found what she termed "protective communication" toward parents by teenagers wanting and needing to protect them. It is possible that similar patterns emerge among adult survivors and those close to them. The potential role for professional helpers to provide a space for survivors to explore their fears and anxieties may therefore become even more important as time goes on.

Conclusion

This chapter has aimed to explore the research and theoretical basis for understanding the psychological and psychosocial issues surrounding sperm banking following a cancer diagnosis, though the findings may be applicable to other health conditions. It has drawn primarily on the experience of teenagers and included reference to adults from time to time.

It has suggested that the impact of fertility impairment on survivors is increasingly recognized as a significant long-term effect of cancer. When remission appears to be well established, survivors talk of the difficulty of "moving on" when reproductive choice has been removed. The provision of sperm banking has the potential to ameliorate this and reduce levels of distress by affording "hopefulness" through potentially offering an alternative route through which to exercise reproductive choice. Where treatment is not successful and men move into palliative care, sperm banking may carry a different, and equally important, type of emotional and social significance as well as offering the potential for achieving fatherhood (including posthumously). Attention to the physical and emotional context of sperm banking is crucial to avoid the risk of inducing lasting distress through participation in the process itself.

References

Arthur, V.A.M. (1995). Written patient information: a review of the literature. *Journal of Advanced Nursing*, **21**, 1081–6.

Bahadur, G., Whelan, J., Ralph, D. & Hindmarsh, P. (2001). Gaining consent to freeze spermatozoa from adolescents with cancer: legal, ethical and practical aspects. *Human Reproduction*, **16**, 188–93.

Bauld, C., Anderson, V. & Arnold, J. (1998). Psychosocial aspects of adolescent cancer survival. *Journal of Paediatric Child Health*, **34**, 120–6.

Beaver, K. & Luker, K. (1997). Readability of patient information booklets for women with breast cancer. *Patient Education and Counselling*, **31**, 95–102.

Bennett, P. (2000). *Introduction to Clinical Psychology*. Buckingham, UK: Open University Press.

Blacklay, A., Eiser, C. & Ellis, A. (1998). Development and evaluation of an information booklet for adult survivors of cancer in childhood. *Archives of Disease in Childhood*, **78**, 340–4.

Broome, M.E. & Allegretti, C. (2001). Letters to the Editor: Adolescent cancer patients: sperm storage, consent and emotion and reply by Gulam Bahadur. *Human Reproduction*, **16**, 2473–7.

Charmaz, K. (1994). Identity dilemmas of chronically ill men. *Sociological Quarterly*, **35**, 269–88.

Coleman, J.C. & Hendry, L.B. (1999). *The Nature of Adolescence*, 3rd edn. London: Routledge.

Cooke, I.D. (2003). A strategy for fertility services for survivors of childhood cancer – report of a multidisciplinary working group convened by the BFS. *Human Fertility*, **6**, A1–A40.

Coulson, C., Kershaw, H., Radford, J. & Larcher, V. (2001). Semen collection from young cancer patients. *Human Fertility*, **4**, 131–4.

Crawshaw, M.A., Glaser, A.W., Hale, J.K., Phelan, L. & Sloper, P. (2003). *A Study of the Decision Making Process Surrounding Sperm Storage for Adolescent Minors within Paediatric Oncology*. Available from Department of Social Policy & Social Work, University of York, York YO10 5DD, UK.

Crawshaw, M.A., Glaser, A.W., Hale, J.K. & Sloper, P. (2004). Professionals' views on the issues and challenges arising from providing a fertility preservation service through sperm banking to teenage males with cancer. *Human Fertility*, **7**, 23–30.

Culley, L., Rapport, F., Katbamna, S., Johnson, M. & Hudson, N. (2004). *A Study of Provision of Infertility Services to South Asian Community*. Final Report prepared for NHS Executive Policy and Practice Research and Development Programme, Leicester, UK: De Montfort University.

Daniel, B. & Wassell, S., (2002). *Adolescence: Assessing and Promoting Resilience in Vulnerable Children 3*. London: Jessica Kingsley.

Edwards, J.L., Gibson, F., Richardson, A., Sepion, B. & Ream, E. (2003). Fatigue in adolescents with and following a cancer diagnosis: developing an evidence base for practice. *European Journal of Cancer*, **39**, 2671–80.

Eiser, C. (1998) Practitioner review: long term consequences of childhood cancer. *Journal of Child Psychology and Psychiatry*, **39**, 621–33.

Fallowfield, L., Ford, S. & Lewis, S. (1995). No news is not good news: information preferences of patients with cancer. *Psycho-Oncology*, **4**, 197–202.

Faulkner, A., Peace, G. & O'Keefe, C. (1995). *When a Child has Cancer*. London: Chapman & Hall.

Fraser, C., Balen, R. & Fielding D. (2006). The views of the next generation: an exploration of priorities for adulthood and the meaning of parenthood amongst 10–16 year olds. In R. Balen & M. Crawshaw, eds., *Sexuality and Fertility Issues in Ill Health and Disability: From Early Adolescence to Adulthood*. London: Jessica Kingsley, pp. 33–48.

Green, D., Galvin, H. & Horne, B. (2003). The psycho-social impact of infertility on young male cancer survivors: a qualitative investigation. *Psycho-Oncology*, **12**, 141–52.

Grinyer, A. (2002). *Cancer in Young Adults: Through Parents' Eyes*. Buckingham, UK: Open University Press.

Heiney, S.P. (1989). Adolescents with cancer: sexual and reproductive issues. *Cancer Nursing*, **12**, 95–101.

Kameny, R.R. & Bearison, D.J. (2002). Cancer narratives of adolescents and young adults: a quantitative and qualitative analysis. *Children's Health Care*, **31**, 143–73.

Kubler-Ross, E. (1997). *On Death and Dying*. New York, NY: Touchstone.

Langton, H. (2000). *The Child with Cancer: Family-centred Care in Practice*. Edinburgh, UK: Balliere Tindall.

Lee, S. (1996). *Counselling in Male Infertility*. Oxford, UK: Blackwell Science Ltd.

Lozowoski, S.L. (1993). Views of childhood cancer survivors. *Cancer*, **71**, 3354–7.

Malus, M., LaChance, P.A., Lamy, L., Macaulay, A. & Vanasse, M. (1987). Priorities in adolescent health care: the teenager's viewpoint. *Journal of Family Practice*, **25**, 159–62.

Marik, J.J. (2004). Live birth with sperm cyopreserved for 21 years. *Human Reproduction*. **19**, 2680.

Mason, M.-C. (1993). *Male Infertility – Men Talking*. London: Routledge.

Miller, S., Schroeder, C. & Mangan, C. (1996). Application of the monitoring process model to coping with severe long-term medical threats. *Health Psychology*, **15**, 216–25.

Monach, J.H. (1993). *Childless No Choice: The Experience of Involuntary Childlessness*. London: Routledge.

Moynihan, C. (1998). Theories of masculinity. *British Medical Journal*, **317**, 1072–5.

Moynihan, C., Bliss, J.M., Davidson, J., Burchell, L. & Horwich, A. (1998). Evaluation of adjuvant psychological therapy in patients with testicular cancer: randomised controlled trial. *British Medical Journal*, **316**, 429–35.

Neville, K. (1998). The relationships among uncertainty, social support, and psychological distress in adolescents recently diagnosed with cancer. *Journal of Pediatric Oncology Nursing*, **15**, 37–46.

Neville, K. (2000). *Mature Beyond Their Years: The Impact of Cancer on Adolescent Development*. Pittsburgh, PA: Oncology Nursing Press.

Oakley, A., Bendelow, G., Barnes, J., Buchanan, M. & Husain, O.A. (1995). Health and cancer prevention: knowledge and beliefs of children and young people. *British Medical Journal*, **310**, 1029–33.

Ogden, J. (2001). *Health Psychology: A Text Book*. Buckingham, UK: Open University Press.

Pacey, A. (2003). Sperm you can bank on. *British Medical Journal*, **327**, 1354.

Parkes, C.M. (1996). *Bereavement: Studies of Grief in Adult Life*. London: Tavistock.

Parkes, C.M., Laungani, P. & Young, B. (2003). *Death and Bereavement across Cultures*. London: Routledge.

Puukko, L.R., Hirvonen, E., Aalberg, V. *et al.* (1997). Sexuality of young women surviving leukemia. *Archive of Disease in Childhood*, **76**, 197–202.

Roberts, C.S., Turney, M.E. & Knowles, A.M. (1998). Psychosocial issues of adolescents with cancer. *Social Work in Heath Care*, **27**, 3–18.

Ryan, G. (2000). Childhood sexuality: a decade of study. Part 1 – research and curriculum development. *Child Abuse and Neglect*, **24**, 33–48.

Salander, P. & Hamberg, K. (2005). Gender differences in patients' written narratives about being diagnosed with cancer. *PsychoOncology*, **14**, 684–95.

Schover, L.R. (1997). *Sexuality and Fertility after Cancer*. New York, NY: John Wiley & Sons.

Schover, L.R., Rybicki, L.A., Martin, B.A. & Bringelsen, K.S. (1999). Having children after cancer: a pilot survey of survivors' attitudes and experiences. *Cancer*, **86**, 697–709.

Schover, L.R., Brey, K., Lichtin, A., Lipshultz, L.I. & Jeha, S. (2002a). Oncologists' attitudes and practices regarding banking sperm before cancer treatment. *Journal of Clinical Oncology*, **20**, 1890–7.

Schover, L.R., Brey, K., Lichtin, A., Lipshultz, L.I. & Jeha, S. (2002b). Knowledge and experience regarding cancer, infertility, and sperm banking in younger male cancer survivors. *Journal of Clinical Oncology*, **20**, 1880–9.

Self, M. (2006). Becoming a parent – the transition to parenthood where there is preexisting fertility impairment. In R. Balen & M. Crawshaw, eds., *Sexuality and Fertility Issues in Ill health and Disability: From Early Adolescence to Adulthood*. London: Jessica Kingsley. pp. 234–47.

Senanayake, P., Nott, J.H. & Faulkener, K.M. (2001). Adolescent sexual and reproductive health: the challenge for society. *Human Fertility*, **4**, 117–22.

Stead, M.L., Fallowfield, L., Brown, J.M. & Selby, P. (2001). Communication about sexual problems and sexual concerns in ovarian cancer: qualitative study. *British Medical Journal*, **323**, 836–7.

Stroebe, M.S., Stroebe, W.S. & Hanson R.O. (2001). *Handbook of Bereavement*. Cambridge: Cambridge University Press.

The, A-M., Hak, T., Koeter, G. & van der Wal, G. (2000). Collusion in doctor–patient communication about imminent death: an ethnographic study. *British Medical Journal*, **321**, 1376–81.

Wallace, W.H.B. & Walker, D.A. (2001). Conference Consensus Statement: ethical and research dilemmas for fertility preservation in children treated for cancer. *Human Fertility*, **4**, 69–76.

Worden, J.W. (2002). *Grief Counseling and Grief Therapy. A Handbook for the Mental Health Practitioner*, 3rd edn. New York, NY: Springer Publishing Company.

Young, B., Dixon-Woods, M., Windbridge, K. C. & Heney, D. (2003). Managing communication with young people who have a potentially life threatening chronic illness: qualitative study of patients and parents. *British Medical Journal*, **326**, 305.

Zebrack, B. (2006). Young adult cancer survivors: Shaken up. Getting back. Moving on. In R. Balen & M. Crawshaw, eds., *Sexuality and Fertility Issues in Ill health and Disability: From Early Adolescence to Adulthood*. London: Jessica Kingsley, pp. 221–33.

Zebrack, B.J., Zeltzer, L.K., Whitton, J. *et al.* (2002). Psychological outcomes in long-term survivors of childhood leukemia, Hodgkin's disease and non-Hodgkin's lymphoma: a report from the Childhood Cancer Survivor Study. *Pediatrics*, **110**, 42–52.

Zebrack, B.J., Casillas, J., Nohr, L., Adams, H. & Zeltzer, L.K. (2004). Fertility issues for young adult cancer survivors of childhood cancer. *PsychoOncology*, **13**, 689–99.

5 Legal and ethical aspects of sperm banking

Susan Avery

Introduction

Sperm banking is unusual in that it involves patients and practitioners in a medical procedure that does not involve any treatment or physical processes for the individual concerned beyond procurement of the sperm to be banked. The individual then has certain rights over the disposition of this material which do not amount to ownership, yet decisions relating to this material may affect not only on the individual concerned, but his partner, family, and any potential or existing offspring. It is also unusual in that sperm banking in legal minors may, in some countries, be carried out without any requirement for parental consent. In addition, storage of sperm makes it possible for genetic offspring to be conceived after the sperm provider has died. These factors give rise to a number of ethical and legal concerns.

The legal framework under which sperm banking can occur around the world varies considerably, from the situation in the USA where there are no national laws, to that seen in Canada or the UK where specific legislation outlines the parameters under which sperm may be banked. This chapter will draw heavily on UK law to illustrate the complex legal and ethical maze that surrounds sperm banking, using case law where it exists. It is hoped that this will guide readers, in whichever country they reside, to seek more specific guidance concerning the prevailing legal framework that is applicable to them.

Legal frameworks of sperm banking

In the UK, the storage and use of gametes is governed by a piece of legislation that was, at the time of its enactment, unique in the world. The technology of in vitro fertilization (IVF) was first used successfully in the UK (Steptoe & Edwards, 1978), and it was this development that spawned the Warnock Report (Warnock, 1984), which formed the basis of the Human Fertilisation and Embryology Act (1990). The Warnock Committee expressed no apparent concerns about the safety of semen storage, but did highlight the possible legal complications that might arise from prolonged storage of gametes. The Committee was also very concerned with the possible complications of posthumous use of stored sperm, and made a strong recommendation that children conceived after their father's death should be disregarded for the purposes of inheritance and succession.

The Human Fertilisation and Embryology Act (1990) takes account of the Warnock Committee's recommendations, in restricting the uses to which gametes and embryos may be put, and under what circumstances. Within these restrictions, the fate of banked sperm is governed by the need for consent from the gamete providers to any process that might be

Sperm Banking: Theory and Practice, eds. Allan A. Pacey and Mathew J. Tomlinson.
Published by Cambridge University Press. © Cambridge University Press 2009.

carried out using their living gametes. In other countries with comparable legislation, similar restrictions often apply.

It is important to understand that law is based on permission, rather than compulsion. A consent to bank sperm does not compel a practitioner to do so. Nor does consent to use banked sperm, in the treatment of a particular individual, force that treatment to occur. All the normal criteria for a decision to treat must still apply.

Consent

In many countries consent to sperm banking must be in writing, and must also give details of the gamete provider's wishes in the event of their death or mental incapacitation. In the UK, the consent is limited to legal purposes defined under the Human Fertilisation and Embryology Act (1990), and must be specific: gamete providers must specify, within their consent, the duration of storage, and whether the sperm may be used in treatment, and if so, for or with whom, or whether it may be used in research. The 1990 Act also requires clear consent to storage and use, so that consent to one does not imply consent to the other. In theory an individual could consent to storage without making any provisions for use. If consent to future use is given, then a general consent to use in treatment of a named individual is not sufficient to allow use of the sperm in IVF or intracytoplasmic sperm injection (ICSI), as there must be specific consent to the creation of embryos. Although in the UK statutory consent forms are used for the purposes of recording consent, even in countries without specific national legislation (e.g. the USA) it would seem commonplace for individual sperm banks to have their own contracts or agreements to outline the purposes in which the sperm may be stored and used (see Schuster *et al.*, 2003). However, clearly, such contracts need to be robust if legal challenges are to be avoided.

Rights to sperm

The question arises from time to time as to whether the banked sperm, or rights to banked sperm, can be assigned to another individual, as would be possible with personal property, particularly in the event of loss of capacity or death of the gamete-provider. Steinbock and McClamrock (1994) examined the concept of sperm as property in relation to the case of *Hecht v. Superior Court* (1993), where a man wished to transfer control of his sperm to his lover (Hecht), in order that she could conceive his child after he committed suicide. They concluded that this fell outside the arguments against commodification of body parts, and concerns about the commercialization of reproduction, and that respect for autonomy and privacy in matters of reproduction justified the assignment of rights over sperm in the same way as for other property. Bahadur (2002) points out that, for the purposes of transport across European Union (EU) countries, sperm are classified as goods, and therefore unavoidably become property for this purpose. Thus, in the UK, sperm may be property when traveling, but the constraints placed on their use by the Human Fertilisation and Embryology Act (1990) prevents the transfer of rights as for other property, as the existence or non-existence of the appropriate specific consent will ultimately govern the fate of the gametes. This includes consent to export (HFEA, 1991b).

All in all, the legal provisions mean that individuals consenting to sperm storage need careful counseling about the nature of their consent. Their reproductive future may be governed by the decisions they make at the time that sperm storage is proposed. In the UK, consent may be altered within the bounds of the 1990 Act or withdrawn at any time. However, decisions about the fate of the sperm after the provider's death will have implications for his partner and family, which will be unalterable. This also creates problems if the patient is an adolescent (see below). It may be hard for partners and other family members to understand that their wishes will not have any bearing on the fate of the sperm, unless they are in harmony with those of the gamete-provider. Partners may feel that their wishes and their reproductive futures are jeopardized if a man decides not to store sperm when his fertility is in peril, or if he does not consent to posthumous use. Beyond the issue of posthumous use there is also the question of consenting to the possible creation of embryos, and often there is no time for the level of counseling infertility patients usually receive before embarking on assisted conception treatment, when cytotoxic therapy is urgently needed. Pragmatism will often argue in favor of storing the gametes and having these discussions afterward in order that the man can get on with his possibly life-saving treatment, provided he has been given the necessary information in order to make the initial decisions about storage. Nevertheless, counseling should be made available, and not only at the time of storage, but also on an ongoing basis during the storage period. On another practical note, it is essential that sperm bank staff receive thorough training in the completion of legal forms and associated law and regulations.

How long can sperm be stored?

The Warnock Committee recognized that from a biological perspective sperm could be banked indefinitely, or at least for a longer period of time than would be needed to satisfy the needs of patients. It did, however, recommend a five-yearly review for the purposes of: reviewing the wishes of the patients and renewing contact. The Committee did not, however, recommend an absolute limit on storage times, particularly in view of the fact that some patients undergoing cytotoxic therapies might be very young at the time of sperm storage. It was also recognized that it would be unreasonable to expect centers to store material indefinitely. Similarly, a recent European Society for Human Reproduction & Embryology (ESHRE) Task Force on Ethics and Law (2006) concluded that gametes should only be stored until the age at which it is considered acceptable for them to be used for the achievement of a pregnancy, taking into account the welfare of the child and the risks to the pregnant mother. But again, the task force did not recommend an absolute limit.

In the UK, whilst the Human Fertilisation and Embryology Act (1990) specifies a storage period of gametes of 10 years, regulations have been passed which allow for men under the age of 45 to store their sperm until their 55th birthday if their fertility has been permanently impaired (HFEA, 1991a). This gives adequate time for most men to complete their families. However, other countries have been less generous. For example, the 1988 Spanish law governing assisted reproduction techniques (reviewed by Peinado & Russell, 1990) only allowed sperm to be banked for a maximum period of five years, although a later revision to the law in May 2006 (Law 14/2006 in the Spanish BOE [Boietin Oficial del Estrade]) now allows for sperm to be stored until the end of an individual's reproductive life, although interestingly this is not defined by a precise age (Anna Veiga, personal communication). By contrast, in Austria sperm may only be banked for two years under the Austrian Act on Procreative Medicine (1992). Clearly, this would preclude any male who is not in a relationship at the time of his diagnosis and treatment from any reasonable chance of becoming a father using banked sperm.

In Sweden, sperm storage for fertility preservation is not tightly regulated. There are, however, regulations governing the use of donated gametes, and this has led to confusion, as some clinicians have interpreted these rules as though they apply to all cryopreserved sperm. In particular, couples should have a likely life expectancy to coincide at least with the 18th birthday of any resulting child. This, when mistakenly applied, causes serious problems for oncology patients, as clinicians may refuse to use such stored sperm in treatment without evidence that the patient is likely to survive another 19 years! (Lars Bjorndahl, personal communication).

Contact tracing

In countries, such as the UK, where sperm may be banked for extended periods of time (e.g. up to 40 years if the patient was 15 at the time of banking and his fertility remained impaired), sperm banks are presented with problems in maintaining contact with patients who have no obligation or reason to contact the sperm bank unless they wish to use the samples. This means that limits on storage may therefore be set locally and depend on funding arrangements in place. The Human Fertilisation and Embryology Authority (HFEA) *Code of Practice* (HFEA, 2007) states that sperm banks should carry out reviews once every two years for the general purposes of audit but also to review the purposes and duration of storage, and check what action needs to be taken. Furthermore, the sperm bank is expected to operate a bring-forward system so that there is sufficient notice of the end of the statutory storage period in each case, and to endeavor to maintain contact with the providers of stored gametes in order to give them reasonable notice of the end of the storage period so that they have time to make decisions and to have access to appropriate information and advice.

Practically, sperm banks are expected to take reasonable measures to maintain contact with patients. Patients who do not respond to letters, and cannot be contacted in any other way, may often be traced by means that do not compromise confidentiality. However, it is not unusual for sperm banks to be unable to contact patients. This may be because of a change of address, a conscious decision not to respond, or because the patient has died. Lack of response leaves sperm banks with a dilemma. If they have no evidence that the patient is deceased, or if he has consented to posthumous storage sperm banks can keep the sperm in storage until the end of the legal storage period. This leads to problems of cost and storage capacity, and banks may have contractual arrangements with patients who have paid to store their sperm, specifying that the material will be removed from storage if the patient does not maintain contact and/or pay the storage fees. Such contracts need careful legal scrutiny, and this is a much more difficult issue when the storage has been funded by a health service, as the contract may be between the funding body and the sperm bank. Banks should take professional legal advice on all such agreements. Even with contracts in place, there will be fear that a patient will reappear after his samples have been disposed of, having failed to maintain contact for some reason outside of his control, such as illness.

Another problem sperm banks often face is that of establishing whether a patient is dead or alive. In the UK, if a bank maintains samples in storage after the patient's death, where there is not consent to posthumous storage, they are technically in breach of the Human Fertilisation and Embryology Act (1990) even if they had no means of knowing that a patient has died. However, the regulatory authority is likely to treat centers sympathetically in these circumstances if they have complied with the *Code of Practice* (HFEA, 2007), and taken reasonable steps to contact the patient. Nevertheless many sperm banks often store sperm for uncontactable patients at significant expense, in order to prevent the problems that might occur as a result of disposing of them. There are no simple solutions to this, but clearly it is essential that patients are made well aware of their obligations and the risks they run by failing to keep in touch.

Sperm storage for minors and adolescents

Since sperm is usually stored under circumstances where fertility is under threat (see Chapter 2) the preservation of fertility is, therefore, an issue, not only for adults, but for children and adolescents.

Sperm banking may be carried out for almost any postpubertal male who is able to provide a sample or where one can be surgically recovered (Chapter 6). Given that only the provider of gametes can give consent to storage, we have a situation where a clinical procedure must, if it is to be carried out, be consented to by a minor. The law in the UK does not allow for substitution of consent with regard to sperm banking, that is, parents cannot consent of behalf of their child. However, sperm freezing is distinguished from medical treatment in general in that nothing is actually done to the patient in most instances. It is also distinguished in that the procedure has implications for the future for both parents and child, beyond the life of the child himself. In general, children in the UK who are under the age of 16 can give legally valid consent to medical treatment if the clinician believes they are competent to make a sensible informed decision (*Gillick v. Norfolk and Wisbech Area Health Authority*, 1985; Age of Legal Capacity (Scotland) Act 1991 s2,(4); Alderson, 2000; Hedley, 2000). The 1989 Children Act (Children's Act, 1989) and equivalent Acts for Scotland and Northern Ireland allow for children to "refuse medical or psychiatric examination" if deemed competent.

The need for patients to understand all issues in order to give informed consent is clearly essential, regardless of the age or maturity of the patient. Bahadur *et al.* (2001) point out that here are many unknowns, including sperm quality pre- and postthaw, which prevent consent to sperm storage from ever being fully informed. They also point out that consent is required, not only to storage but also to subsequent treatment using the sperm, and the fate of the sperm in the event of the patient's death. In the case of minors there can clearly be no informed consent to use in treatment as they will have no partner who can be named and sperm cannot be considered as property (see above). Having no partner may also prevent adult patients from making these decisions, and in such situations patients can only consent to storage, and make clear their wishes in the event of death. Considering the circumstances this is a tough call and the complexities involved have been discussed in Chapter 4.

The Gillick case (*Gillick v. W. Norfolk and Wisbech Area Health Authority*, 1985) provides a model that is now commonly used in the UK to determine the competence of a minor to make decisions in relation to his or her treatment. Victoria Gillick, a mother of five girls, sought a declaration that prescribing contraception to under-16s was illegal in that it would not only involve the offence of encouraging sex with a minor, but would also amount to treatment without consent, as the power of consent would be vested in the parent. The House of Lords held that minors could consent to treatment in some circumstances, and that, in such circumstances the parent would not have the power of veto. Lord Scarman proposed that the test, subsequently known as the test of Gillick competency, should be whether the child had sufficient "understanding and intelligence" to enable them to comprehend the medical treatment that is proposed. Gillick competency is now the measure used to decide whether a child is able to give consent to sperm storage. Section 6.4.2 of the *Code of Practice* (HFEA, 2007) points storage centers to the definition of Gillick competence as laid down by the General Medical Council (GMC) in its ethical considerations guidelines (GMC, 1998):

You must assess a child's capacity to decide whether to consent or refuse investigation or treatment before you provide it. In general, a competent child will be able to understand the nature, purpose, and possible consequences of the proposed investigation or treatment, as well as the consequences of non-treatment.

That there is an emphasis on nontreatment, or in this case, failure to bank sperm, is important. The child will be immediately aware of the issues that might put them off proceeding with storage, and the positive consequences of storage may seem remote. The consequences of failing to store should be made very clear.

Determining the ability to make wise, autonomous decisions is not one that can be made easily on brief acquaintance. Bahadur *et al.* (2001) suggest a process whereby the young patient is well informed before referral to the sperm bank, and that he should then have an opportunity to become familiar with the staff and the environment, and to establish a rapport with the sperm banking personnel. This is, of course, ideal, but in reality there is often urgency about storage that means there is insufficient time, and the referring clinician may well be far more concerned with the patient's survival than preserving his fertility (see Chapter 3). Another problem with early adolescents is their vulnerability to external pressures. Should they feel that they do not wish to proceed with sperm banking they may well come under pressure from their parents who may be concerned, not only that the child is making the wrong decision for its own sake, but also for the loss of their potential grandchildren. On the other hand, it might be considered tragic for a child to turn down the opportunity to bank sperm because he is embarrassed by the process (see Chapter 4).

Particular issues may arise if the patient is unable to produce a sample by masturbation so that surgical sperm retrieval needs to be considered (see Chapter 6), or if the parents disagree with the child's decision. Foreman (1999) proposes a "family rule" for consent, whereby informed consent in children is regarded as shared between the children and their families, the balance being determined by implicit, developmentally based negotiations between child and parent. This may take some pressure off the child, but will not solve the problems that arise when the child's wishes are in conflict with those of his parents.

Practitioners dealing with these situations should consider giving the child an opportunity to express his views in the absence of the parents, if they sense an element of conflict, but it is also necessary to consider carefully who should have such discussions with the child. In practice, time is often an unaffordable luxury, and the balance between allowing sufficient time for counseling and decision-making is balanced with the urgency of commencing cytotoxic therapy. Nevertheless, it is essential that all staff concerned with sperm banking are aware of the specific issues that affect young people and are able to deal with the situation in a highly sensitive way, giving thought to the feelings of both children and parents. Early dialog and communication between the pediatric team and the sperm bank is therefore vital (see Chapter 3).

Posthumous use of stored sperm

Posthumous use of sperm cannot be considered an awkward consequence of sperm banking, but rather it is a defined purpose for sperm storage. It caused the Warnock Committee (Warnock, 2002) the greatest concern and has recently been reviewed by the ESHRE Task Force on Ethics and Law (2006), revealing wide differences in national laws concerning the subject. Interestingly, the ESHRE report identified that there was no consensus among the different religions, with Roman Catholics rejecting it because it separates human reproduction from sexual intercourse and implies insemination of a single woman. Posthumous conception is forbidden in a number of countries, including Germany and Italy. It is no surprise that Italian law stipulates that both parents-to-be must be alive at the time of treatment, although, interestingly, if the man's death occurs between the time of fertilization and implantation, the process is not interrupted and all fertilized embryos must be transferred to the woman's womb (Boggio, 2005) as embryo storage is not allowed. By contrast, Islam rejects posthumous reproduction because it takes place after the end of the marital term, whereas Jewish law permits posthumous procreation (ESHRE Task Force on Ethics and Law, 2006).

In the UK, the Human Fertilisation and Embryology Act (1990) contains some specific provisions relating to posthumous storage and use, most notably the need for written consent. However, while posthumous conception may be permissible within this frame-work, its desirability and acceptability are different issues that arouse strong feelings. As well as the needs or wishes of the prospective parents, the interests and welfare of any potential child must be considered. The advisability of posthumous use of sperm may also be affected by individual circumstances, and this may conflict with the wishes of the deceased. From time to time the wishes of the deceased may also be in conflict with those of the living, and the views of the medical practitioners involved may further complicate the matter.

Possibly the most notorious case in Europe relating to intervention in human repro-duction is that of *Regina v. Human Fertilisation and Embryology Authority ex parte Blood* (1997). This case embraces many of the legal and ethical issues relating to sperm storage and posthumous use.

Mr. and Mrs. Blood had been contemplating fertility treatment, although they had not embarked on it, when Stephen Blood contracted viral meningitis and as a consequence was placed on a life-support machine, with no hope of recovery. At his wife's request, semen was collected via rectal electro-ejaculation (see Chapter 6) and was banked. Under the circumstances it was impossible to obtain his consent, either to the rectal electro-ejaculation or the sperm banking. The practitioners involved sought the advice of the HFEA, and it would appear that both sides considered the legal position to be unclear, and the procedure went ahead on the basis that deciding against collecting sperm at this point would be an irreversible decision. It does not seem that a great deal of consideration was given to the position in relation to the rectal electro-ejaculation without consent.

Diane Blood maintained that she and Stephen had discussed the question of post-humous conception and that he had verbally and informally given his consent. It would appear that the HFEA advised the clinicians to go ahead as this was, in legal terms, unexplored territory. It is to be supposed that this was considered the humane course of action. However, on the face of it, it is hard to see why this situation ever arose. The UK Human Fertilisation and Embryology Act (1990) is clear on the need for written consent to sperm storage. No such consent existed, nor was there any opportunity to obtain it.

It was when Diane Blood sought permission from the HFEA to use the sperm in treatment that the legal arguments were explored as permission was refused. Again, the 1990 Act is clear. Gametes cannot be used in treatment without written consent and embryos cannot be created under any circumstances, without consent. Mrs. Blood also sought permission to take the sperm abroad, as EU law entitled her to seek medical treatment in any EU country. Permission was refused. The HFEA has powers of discretion to allow export of gametes, but here they were dealing with gametes that were illegally stored, and where there was no consent for use, or to export, for that matter. Diane Blood sought a judicial review of the decisions and was refused, on the grounds that the HFEA had no discretion in this matter, as the requirements for consent to storage and use were clearly laid down in the Human Fertilisation and Embryology Act (1990).

Mrs. Blood appealed on the grounds that s4(1)b of the 1990 Act allowed treatment of a couple together without written consent, and also on the basis that European Community (EC) law allowed her to seek treatment in any EU country, and that the decision of the HEFA not to allow export of the sperm was, in effect, an infringement of that right. The Court of Appeal upheld the decision of the HFEA not to allow the sperm to be used in the UK, but also said that the Authority should reconsider its decision not to allow export. The HFEA did so, and subsequently allowed the export of Stephen Blood's sperm to Belgium where Diane was treated successfully.

The Human Fertilisation and Embryology Act (1990) makes it a requirement, not only for there to be written consent to sperm storage, but also for there to be a written statement as to what should be done with the gametes if the person who has given the consent dies (Sch 3, para 2). The sperm may then only continue to be stored or used, in line with the existing consents (para 2(1) and para 5(1) and (3)). Thus it is the wishes of the deceased that controls the fate of the sperm, rather than any desires of the living. The Court of Appeal made it clear that, in Stephen Blood's case, since no written consent existed the storage had taken place illegally, and that, therefore, a criminal offence had been committed by the license-holder under s41(2)b. However, no action was taken against him. In relation to this Lord Woolf explained it as follows:

There is . . . no question of any prosecution being brought in the circumstances of this case, and no possible criticism can be made of the fact that storage has taken place because Professor Cooke of the IRT was acting throughout in close consultation with the Authority in a perfectly bona fide manner, in an unexplored legal situation where humanity dictated that the sperm was taken and preserved first, and the legal argument followed. From now on, however, the legal situation will be different as these proceedings will clarify the legal position. Because this judgement makes it clear that the sperm of Mr Blood has been preserved and stored when it should not have been, this case raises issues as to the lawfulness of the use and export of sperm which should never arise again.

This last statement is crucial to the final outcome of this case and, as we shall see, leads to an outcome that might be considered humane, if not legally very satisfactory.

The question arises as to whether there are any circumstances that would have allowed the sperm to be used within the bounds of the Human Fertilisation and Embryology Act (1990). Mrs. Blood's case was argued on the basis that such a circumstance did exist in the exception under s4(1)(b). This allows for couples to be treated "together" using the male partner's sperm, without the need for written consent and outside of the terms of any license. This led the Court of Appeal to examining the meaning of "treatment together" and whether a couple could be considered to be undergoing treatment together if one partner was deceased. The 1990 Act makes specific provision for posthumous use of sperm, not only in defining the paternal status of the deceased (s28(6), but also in that, under s2(2)(b) of schedule 3, written consent to storage must give instructions as to what is to be done with the sperm if the provider of the gametes dies. This implies that posthumous use of sperm is to be carried out under the terms of a license, and with consent. Overriding this is that fact that posthumous use will, in the vast majority of cases, require storage to take place, and there is no exception defined under the 1990 Act to the need for written consent to storage. The exception under s4(1)(b) would seem to apply only to circumstances where sperm is used immediately, and in such a situation there is no doubt that the couple are being treated together. Thus, if one partner is deceased a couple cannot be considered to as being treated together for the purposes of the 1990 Act.

The second part of Mrs. Blood's appeal was that she should be allowed treatment in another EU country, and that the HFEA should allow export of the sperm to enable this to take place under the provisions of s24(4). This section gives the HFEA discretion as to the conditions that would permit export in any particular case. The HFEA (1991b) general directions state that the gamete provider must give specific consent to export. Articles 59 and 60 of the EC Treaty state that citizens of the community have a right to receive medical treatment in any member state. It was argued on behalf of Mrs. Blood that refusal to allow export of the sperm constituted an infringement of this right. The counterargument put on behalf of the HFEA was that there was no infringement as all that was being refused was leave to export the sperm, and Mrs. Blood could receive any treatment she wanted in Europe.

However, as Lord Woolf puts it, this "approach does not make sufficient allowance for the reality of the situation. It is to this which regard has to be had when considering the entitlement to the provision of services under Article 59. The refusal to permit exports prevents Mrs Blood having the only treatment which she wants."

The Court allowed the appeal in relation to the export decision on the basis that the HFEA had failed to have sufficient regard to Mrs. Blood's right to treatment in another member state, and that the HFEA had been wrongly concerned that a precedent would be created that would allow the law to be circumvented in future cases. The Court had made it clear that such a case could not arise again under the existing legislation, and therefore this concern was spurious. However, the HFEA would still be free to make its own decision regarding export, on the basis that it was clear that the above considerations had been taken into account.

It might be said that, by allowing the export of Mr. Blood's sperm, the HFEA might be said to have acted ultimately in the spirit of the law rather than to the letter, considering that, as Lord Woolf puts it, "the evidence that Mrs. Blood puts forward that her husband would have given his consent in writing if he had had the opportunity to do so is compelling." This relies on the evidence of others as to the wishes of an individual who is unable to represent themselves (as a result of being dead) in a situation where the representatives have, themselves powerful interests, and is in conflict with the Human Fertilisation and Embryology (1990) Act and the HFEA (1991b) general directions. This leads us to consider the way in which the sperm was obtained. Lord Woolf rightly separates the issue of legality of storage and use of the sperm from the manner in which it was obtained, which is not dealt with by the 1990 Act. This would have been a battery at the very least should anyone have chosen to press charges. The procedure could not be said to have been carried out to preserve life, or even the quality of life in this case. Rectal electroejaculation has only one clear aim, and Stephen Blood's life expectancy at this time was virtually nil. It has been suggested that this has an ethical equivalence with rape (McLachlan & Swales, 2003).

To carry out any medical or surgical treatment of an individual when that individual is incapable of giving consent can only be justified on the basis that it is in the patient's best interests, either in terms of saving their life, or in terms of their quality of life. It seems reasonable to argue than an individual who has been given no possibility of survival has no best interests, and thus any procedure carried out was in the best interests of a third party. Susan Bewley comments in Swinn et al. (1998) that "it is a shame that in the public furore about denying Mrs Blood access to the sperm sample once it existed, the initial wrong of taking it was overlooked" and suggested that it "must be hard in an urgent, emotionally charged situation to deny a wife's wishes, but unless there is the clearest guidance, there should be a complete moratorium on such sperm retrieval. Doctors must find the courage to say no to assaulting vulnerable, brain dead patients."

She was commenting as a result of a case where a patient who had been declared brain-dead had an orchidectomy after his wife produced a typed note indicating that, in the event of his death he wished sperm to be stored to enable his wife to have his children. It was signed and dated, but there were concerns nevertheless. Bewley points out that he may have consented to sperm storage and use, but not to the orchidectomy. While the method employed in Stephen Blood's case (rectal electro-ejaculation) may seem less drastic, this too was an invasive procedure and was carried out on his person without his consent. This is not the place for a detailed discourse on the issues of common law and best interests in relation to medical procedures, but it would seem reasonable to state that the person whose best interests are being served by such procedures is the wife or partner and not the patient. Thus it would not be right to ask them to make a decision on the patient's behalf or give consent.

The development of assisted conception has led increasingly to situations where the relative reproductive rights of males and females come into conflict. Women may bear children in the case of absence or death of their partner without any need for a third party to become involved biologically. This is obviously not the case for men. This possibility seems to give greater weight to the desires and rights of the female. There was great public sympathy for Natalie Evans, just as there was for Diane Blood, in a recent case involving a male partner's withdrawal of consent to the use of embryos (Dyer, 2007). In neither case does there seem to have been public concern for the rights of the men. This seems to stem from the greater emphasis on the female drive for maternity and from the social, philosophical, and sentimental views of motherhood that pervade society, rather than any male feelings about reproduction. Logically, there is no reason why a male's right to decide when, with whom, and under what circumstances he should procreate should in any way be subjugated by the female's rights.

In the UK both the male and female rights are protected to the same extent by the Human Fertilisation and Embryology Act (1990). With the exception of Stephen Blood, this legislation has so far protected the rights of the male, and the Blood case, in the end, served to reinforce this. However, the issues of obtaining sperm when there is no consent to the procedure remain, and will doubtless arise again as such situations occur in the event of unexpected death rather than in cases of long-term illnesses where storage may be planned, and consent dealt with accordingly.

In a recent consultation document on reform of the 1990 Act, the question was raised as to whether it should be legal to store sperm where the provider was incapable of giving consent, and where the sperm had been obtained or extracted legally (i.e. without the patient's consent). It is hard to envisage a situation where a patient would be capable of giving consent to obtaining sperm, but incapable of consenting to storage. It is unlikely that consent to one would be taken without consent to the other. The only other possibility would be if the patient was unable to give consent to obtaining sperm, but it was considered to be in their best interests (*F v. West Berkshire Health Authority*, 1989; *Airedale NHS Trust v. Bland*, 1993). However, unless the state that rendered them incapable of giving consent also threatened their fertility it would be difficult again to envisage a scenario that fits this.

Nearly 20 years after the Warnock Committee was convened, Baroness Warnock expressed sympathy with Mrs. Blood, and states that she felt this was an unnecessarily strict application of the rules, and seems to lay some responsibility for the decision at the feet of the then Chair of the HFEA who had strong feelings about posthumous conception (Warnock, 2002). It must be understood that this was never the HFEA's decision to make. The entire process was illegal under the Human Fertilisation and Embryology Act (1990), if not under common law. We may all feel sympathy toward the childless and the bereaved. Nevertheless, hard cases make bad law, as the maxim runs. The question of using the sperm should never have arisen since its procurement and storage had both been illegal. In addition, to allow its use would have been to negate the reproductive rights of the gentleman concerned. There is no evidence that Mr. Blood would have been happy to have his child conceived after his death. There is certainly no evidence that he would have been happy to have been physically treated in this way when he was on the point of death.

One might also consider that, had the argument in relation to the exception under 4(1)b been accepted, Diane Blood's problems would not have been resolved, as this would only have applied to artificial insemination, and not IVF or ICSI, as the law is also clear in relation to the need for consent for creation of embryos using an individual's gametes. A further consequence of the Blood case was the change in UK law relating to legal paternity after posthumous conception. The Human Fertilisation and Embryology (Deceased Fathers) Bill was passed in September 2003 and, although it does not affect the issue of inheritance or other legal rights, it does allow the deceased father to be recorded in the birth register. However, prospectively, a separate consent is required from the male, which needs to be completed if a man storing sperm consents to posthumous use. This Act came into being after a long campaign by Diane Blood to enable her deceased husband's name to appear on the birth certificates of her children.

The question of posthumous conception by a surrogate in order to provide grieving parents with a grandchild has also been raised (Fraser, 1999). In this case Lance Smith died as a result of injuries sustained in a car crash. Before his death sperm was surgically retrieved and stored at the request of his parents, who produced a note written by their son expressing his wish that his fiancée be treated with his sperm in the event of his death. When his partner decided not to go ahead with insemination his parents sought permission to have the sperm released to treat a surrogate, having produced a second written consent that implied that this was also their son's wish. The treatment did not take place. However, the views expressed by the parents in the press made it clear that it was their wishes that they were concerned with rather than their son's. Smith's mother told the press that disposal of the sperm would be like her son dying all over again. In this case any child would have been born for a clear purpose, that is, to console the parents for their loss. Thus there would be major concerns for such a child, centering on the grandparent's expectation, as well as the legal and social complications surrounding the status of such a child.

A second, less well-publicized, case that explored issues relating to posthumous use of sperm relates at least as much to the ethical views of the clinicians involved, and their ability to influence patients (*Centre for Reproduction v. Mrs. U*, 2002). In this case the management of the clinic concerned expressed clear disapproval of posthumous conception in their literature, and, although the male partner had originally consented to posthumous use of his sperm, he was persuaded to retract this consent by a member of the clinic staff. His wife, wishing to be treated after his death, which was sudden and unexpected, claimed that he had changed his consent as a result of undue influence. In the end, while it was clear that some influence was brought to bear, Mr. U made the decision to change his consent of his own free will. In the final decision of the Court of Appeal, Lady Justice Hale defines the natural response to all of these cases:

We can only guess at the feelings of someone who has suffered as Mrs. U has suffered, but we can sympathize and even empathize with them. There is a natural human temptation to try to bend the law so as to give her what she wants and what she truly believes her husband would have wanted. But we have to resist it.

Welfare of the child

A further issue raised by posthumous conception is that of the welfare of the potential child. This concept, as applied to assisted-conception patients generally, is a vague one, and has never been particularly well defined either in law (Human Fertilisation and Embryology Act, 1990) or in expert guidance (ESHRE Task Force on Ethics and Law et al., 2006). In relation to posthumous conception there are some clear points to consider.

Clearly, the child will be brought into a single-parent family. Depending on the emphasis put on the need for a father, it may be considered that the Human Fertilisation and Embryology Act (1990) is contradictory, allowing posthumous conception, while giving particular weight to the need for a father. The impact on any child of being born into a single-parent household may not be as significant in terms of support, family relationships, and opportunities for development as other social factors (Golombok, 1998). In addition, it has been pointed out (Strong & Schinfeld, 1984; Robertson, 1994; Strong, 1997; Strong et al., 2000) that the acts that are harmful to the child are the very acts that bring them into being. In this context, a harmful action is one which results in the individual being worse off than he or she would otherwise have been (Feinberg, 1984). Thus, to argue that postmortem insemination causes harm to the resulting child implies that they would have been better off not existing. It is not uncommon for children to be brought up by single parents, and in these cases the pregnancies are wanted and planned. Clinics are obliged to make an assessment of factors that might affect the welfare of the child, such as the presence of any extended family support for the mother, the mother's commitment to, and motivation for having the child, and so on. However, it would be difficult, given that posthumous conception is legal, to find truly compelling reasons for refusing treatment on the basis of the welfare of the child, other than those that might inhibit assisted conception treatment generally.

Where there is consent to posthumous use, sperm banks often have strategies for dealing with the matter of posthumous conception that involve the woman waiting a minimum period before having treatment with the sperm. This is intended to give time for reflection, and to be sure that they are not intending to have a child as a way of dealing with their grief, rather than as a continuation of the plans they might have had to have children with their partner. This deals with the one aspect of the welfare of the child that is unique to posthumous sperm storage.

The future

A number of opinions expressed as a result of a recent public consultation on a review of the UK Human Fertilisation and Embryology Act (1990) were related to sperm banking and provide an interesting snapshot of public opinion of the topic (DOH, 2006). The respondents commented on two main themes: consent and posthumous use.

In relation to consent, interestingly, some respondents felt that the need for this to be in writing and taken prior to sperm banking was unnecessarily restrictive, and that account should be taken of witnessed verbal instructions, or of audio or video recordings. The British Medical Association (BMA) stated its belief that storage should be allowed without written consent if an individual is taken ill suddenly, but is expected to recover with impaired fertility. The BMA also believes that taking the gametes could be justified under the doctrine of best interests (presumably on the basis that the man will recover and the ability to have a family will affect his quality of life). The BMA also expresses the view that the wording should be sufficiently broad to include the storage of gametes from children who are unable to give consent, provided someone with parental responsibility is in agreement. Another respondent stated that it should be mandatory to store gametes in the case of childhood cancer, and consent should not be required.

In contrast, others felt that gametes should only ever be stored with the active consent of the donor, and that there are no circumstances in which removal of gametes from a person unable to give consent would be ethical. The need for written consent to the use of gametes also gave rise to a range of views, including that an incapacitated person's gametes could be used if there was sufficient evidence that he would have given consent if he was able, and that sperm could be used without consent if a widow wishes to have a baby. In contrast, one individual felt that the use of gametes without consent could be described as rape.

With regard to posthumous conception, sympathy for widows who wish to have their deceased partner's children was not unusual among the respondents. However, some were concerned that if the man concerned had never expressed any wishes about posthumous conception or sperm storage, there would be a negation of male reproductive rights. Yet another respondent to the consultation says said: "even though it would be 'nice' for someone to have a baby, say, after the death of the father, it isn't in support of the normal and natural way of things." This is, of course, generally true of assisted conception in many people's view. However, it does bring us to the argument as to whether bearing children is a right, that is whether an individual has a right to have child at any price.

Warnock (2002) expresses concerns about this "new rights-based morality," and the confusion of "that which is passionately and deeply wanted with what is a right." Good law should protect an individual's rights over their gametes, even if it is at the expense of the desires of others, and would seem the most reasonable strategy if it is rights we are primarily concerned with. It is to some extent the protection this affords that has allowed the practice of assisted conception in its many forms to flourish around the world.

In 2006, a bill was proposed in New South Wales (Parliament of New South Wales, 2006) that prevented a prisoner suffering from cancer from accessing free sperm storage (which would have been his right prior to conviction). Prisoners would have to pay for such storage, even if the sperm had been stored while they were at liberty. It is unclear whether this is intended as additional punishment, to prevent public outcry at public resources being lavished on wrongdoers, or a eugenic effort in terms of eliminating the "criminal seed" (Rasko, 2006). Thus, while an individual should be allowed to make decisions regarding their reproductive future, where there are options available, there is no doubt that broader public interests will continue to play a role. Technology has delivered a measure of control over human reproduction. Clearly, legislators will need to maintain an ongoing balance between personal desires, rights of the individual, public interest, and the rights and wellbeing of potential children.

Conclusions

Of all the chapters in this book, this is perhaps the one that might date most quickly. This is because new laws can be written relatively quickly, if politicians and parliament so wish, and as a consequence alter the legal landscape of sperm banking in an instant. It is for this reason that this chapter has not focussed on a comparison of sperm banking legislation in different countries, but, rather, has detailed the main ethical concerns those who have written laws have focussed upon. These tend to surround the areas of consent and the possible posthumous use of sperm, although they are obviously not mutually exclusive.

Clearly, some countries do not have specific legislation that covers sperm banking and in those territories professional guidelines and robust contracts need to be in place to protect all parties. It is clearly incumbent on all who are involved in the sperm banking process to be familiar with prevailing legislation in their country and work within it, as well as being sufficiently familiar with the workings of it to advise patients and their families appropriately at the time that any sperm is banked.

References

Age of Legal Capacity (Scotland) Act (1991). Norwich, UK: HMSO Stationery Office.

Airedale NHS Trust v. Bland (1993). 1 All ER 821, [1993]; 12 BMLR 64 (HL).

Alderson, P. (2000). The rise and fall of children's consent to surgery. *Paediatric Nursing*, **12**, 6–8.

Austrian Act on Procreative Medicine Act 275 (1992). May 14.

Bahadur, G. (2001). The Human Rights Act (1998) and its impact on reproductive issues. *Human Reproduction*, **16**, 785–9.

Bahadur, G. (2002). Death and conception. *Human Reproduction*, **17**, 2769–75.

Bahadur, G., Whelan, J., Ralph, D. & Hindmarsh, P. (2001). Gaining consent to freeze spermatozoa from adolescents with cancer: legal and clinical aspects. *Human Reproduction*, **16**, 188–93.

Boggio, A. (2005). Italy enacts new law on medically assisted reproduction. *Human Reproduction*, **20**, 1153–7.

Centre for Reproduction v. Mrs U. (2002). EWHC 36 (Fam).

Children's Act. (1989). London: The Stationery Office.

Department of Health (DOH). (2006). *Report on the Consultation on the Review of the Human Fertilisation and Embryology Act 1990*. London: People, Science and Policy Ltd.

Dyer, C. (2007). Woman loses final round of battle to use her embryos at European Court. *British Medical Journal*, **334**, 818.

European Society for Human Reproduction & Embryology (ESHRE) Task Force on Ethics and Law, Pennings, G., de Wert, G. *et al.* (2006). ESHRE Task Force on Ethics and Law 11: Posthumous assisted reproduction. *Human Reproduction*, **21**, 3050–3.

F v. West Berkshire Health Authority (1989). 2 All ER 545, [1990] 2 AC 1.

Feinberg, J. (1984). *Harm to Others*. Oxford: Oxford University Press.

Foreman, D.M. (1999). The family rule: a framework for obtaining ethical consent for medical interventions from children. *Journal of Medical Ethics*, **25**, 491–6.

Fraser, L. (1999). Our son is dead, but his sperm survives and we must give him the baby he wanted so much. *Mail on Sunday*, December 19.

General Medical Council (GMC). (1998). *Seeking Patient's Consent: The Ethical Considerations*. London: GMC.

Gillick v W. Norfolk and Wisbech Area Health Authority. (1985). All ER, 402.

Golombok, S. (1998). New families, old values: considerations regarding the welfare of the child. *Human Reproduction*, **13**, 2342–7.

Hecht v. Superior Court. (1993). 16 Cal. App. 4th 836, 20 Cal. Rptr. 2d 275 (June).

Hedley, M. (2000). Treating children: whole consent counts? *Current Paediatrics*, **10**, 216–18.

HFEA (1990). Human Fertilisation and Embryology Act 1990. London: The Stationery Office.

HFEA (1991a). The Human Fertilisation and Embryology (Statutory Storage Period) Regulations 1991. Statutory Instruments. No. 1540.

HFEA (1991b). *General Directions 1991/8. Export of Gametes*. London: HFEA.

HFEA (2007). *Code of Practice*, 7th edn. London: HFEA.

McLachlan, H.V. & Swales, J.K., (2003). Posthumous insemination and consent: the continuing, troubling case of Mr. and Mrs. Blood. *Human Reproduction and Genetic Ethics*, **9**, 7–12.

Parliament of New South Wales (2006). Correctional Services. Legislation Amendment Bill 2006.

Peinado, J.A. & Russell, S.E. (1990). The Spanish law governing assisted reproduction techniques: a summary. *Human Reproduction*, **5**, 634–6.

Rasko, J.E.J. (2006). Bill to ban reproduction of inmates with cancer proposed in New South

Wales. *Medical Journal of Australia*, **185**, 575–6.

Regina v. Human Fertilisation and Embryology Authority, ex parte Blood. (1997). 2 All ER 687, 35 BMLR 1, CA.

Robertson, J.A. (1994). *Children of Choice: Freedom and the New Reproductive Technologies*. Princeton, NJ: Princeton University Press.

Schuster, T.G., Hickner-Cruz, K., Ohl, D.A., Goldman, E & Smith, G.D. (2003). Legal considerations for cryopreservation of sperm and embryos. *Fertility and Sterility*, **80**, 61–6.

Steinbock, B. & McClamrock, R. (1994). When is birth is unfair to the child? *The Hastings Center Report* **24**, 15–21.

Steptoe, P.C. & Edwards, R.G. (1978). Birth after the re-implantation of a human embryo. *Lancet*, **2**, 366.

Strong, C. (1997). *Ethics in Reproductive and Perinatal Medicine: A New Framework*. New Haven, CT: Yale University Press.

Strong, C. & Schinfeld, J.S. (1984). The single woman and artificial insemination by donor. *Journal of Reproductive Medicine*, **29**, 293–9.

Strong, C., Gingrich, J.R. & Kutteh, W.H. (2000). Ethics of sperm retrieval after death or persistent vegetative state. *Human Reproduction*, **15**, 739–45.

Swinn, M., Emberton, M., Ralph, D., Smith, M. & Serhal P. (1998). Retrieving semen from a dead patient. *British Medical Journal*, **319**, 57.

Warnock, M. (1984). *Report of the Committee of Inquiry into Human Fertilisation and Embryology*. London: HMSO.

Warnock, M. (2002). *Making Babies*. Oxford, UK: Oxford University Press.

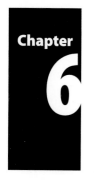

Chapter 6

Methods of sperm retrieval and banking in cancer patients

Sepideh Mehri, Jose Sepulveda, and Pasquale Patrizio

Introduction

Important progress in minimizing the unwanted side effects of therapies such as cytotoxic drug administration or radiotherapy has been achieved by constantly modifying and optimizing the therapeutic regimens, thus enabling many cancer survivors to father children following spontaneous recovery of spermatogenesis (Meistrich, 1999; Brougham *et al.*, 2003). However, the incidence of azoospermia or severe oligozoospermia after cancer treatment remains high, with only about 20–50 percent of these patients having some recovery of spermatogenesis (Shin *et al.*, 2005). Irradiation and chemotherapy each compromise fertility by exerting cytotoxic effects on spermatogonial stem cells and gametogenesis, and the degree of gonadotoxic effect depends on the type, dosage, and duration of the treatment (see Chapter 2).

Besides the toxicity of chemo- and radiotherapy, surgical interventions can also impair future fertility. Retroperitoneal lymph node dissection (RPLND), performed as part of the treatment protocol in testicular cancer patients, may cause ejaculatory dysfunction through emission failure, retrograde ejaculation, or both (Hallak *et al.*, 1999; Lass *et al.*, 1999). Pituitary and adrenal surgery may interfere with the hypothalamic–pituitary–gonadal axis, causing secondary hypogonadism. Inguinal and scrotal surgery may also disrupt the anatomy of the male genital duct system.

Recent advances in assisted reproductive technology have changed the semen parameters that are required for successful fertilization (see Chapter 8). Today, with the technique of intracytoplasmic sperm injection (ICSI), even men with extremely low numbers of sperm can father a child. Because it is difficult to predict the impact of cancer and its therapy on future semen parameters, sperm banking is highly recommended for all patients with malignant disease who wish to preserve their fertility potential (Schover *et al.*, 2002).

Figure 6.1 shows a diagram of the options for obtaining a specimen for banking prior to the commencement of gonadotoxic therapy. While the vast majority of patients will be able to provide a sample by masturbation, for others who cannot or where the masturbatory sample is azoospermic there are other more invasive techniques available which are described throughout this chapter.

Masturbatory ejaculates

The vast majority of sperm banking patients are able to produce an ejaculate by masturbation. The ejaculate should be collected into a suitable sterile specimen container, which is free of contaminants and has been tested to ensure that it is non-toxic to sperm. The container of choice tends to be about 60 mL in volume and manufactured from polypropylene,

Sperm Banking: Theory and Practice, eds. Allan A. Pacey and Mathew J. Tomlinson.
Published by Cambridge University Press. © Cambridge University Press 2009.

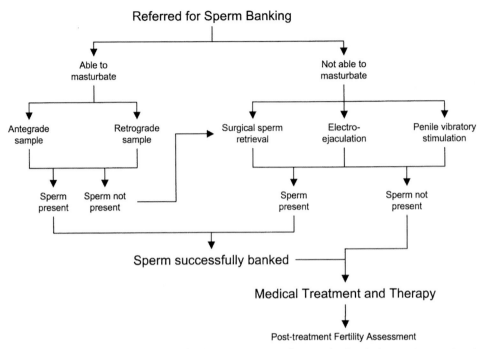

Figure 6.1 Diagram showing the options for obtaining a specimen for sperm banking before starting gonadotoxic therapy. Several options for obtaining specimens are available if the male is unable to masturbate.

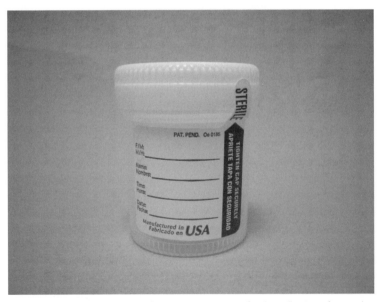

Figure 6.2 A wide-mouthed sterile specimen container for the collection of masturbatory ejaculates.

which is a soft, flexible plastic and unlikely to cause any superficial injury because of sharp edges (Figure 6.2). Adult patients who have a cultural aversion or objection to masturbation, or who simply find it difficult may (if they have a partner) be given the option of using a seminal collection device, which is essentially a non-spermicidal condom, which

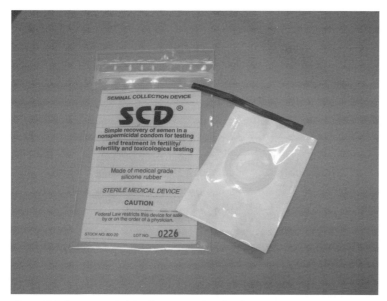

Figure 6.3 A nonspermicidal collection condom for obtaining ejaculates.

can be taken home for collection by intercourse (Figure 6.3). Clearly, the use of these is likely to be restricted by the sperm bank and patients would be required to follow a clear set of guidelines for their use and they may be inappropriate for some patients (e.g. adolescents or those who live a considerable distance away).

There is no written guidance for sperm banks about providing facilities for specimen production either by masturbation or by any other method. Sperm banks must, however, take account of specific patient needs and provide adequate and conducive facilities for patients of varying age, diagnosis, degree of illness, and state of anxiety. Adolescents are understandably often reluctant, anxious, and embarrassed about masturbation, particularly in front of parents and family and in an unfamiliar environment (see Chapter 4). For patients whose illness is making them feel weak or giving them pain, masturbation may be the last thing on their mind, yet many take the pragmatic approach and view the production of a specimen as a "means to an end". Sperm banks should also be mindful of allowing "poorly" inpatients to use their facilities, particularly if unaccompanied by representatives of the medical staff responsible for their care. In these instances it may be more helpful for the hospital department providing their treatment to provide a facility locally which would allow any medical emergency to be handled appropriately and should lead to an increased chance of success. Anxiety in patients can be particularly unhelpful and may increase as their fear from an extraordinary environment is then compounded by an inability to become sexually aroused and the prospect of failure, which represents a threat to future fatherhood.

Although patients may be given the option to produce the specimen at home, on-site facilities must be provided both for inpatients, those who live long distances from the sperm bank, and for those who simply find it more convenient. In short, facilities should:

- Be private and well away from noise.

- Be clean and hygienic, providing facilities for men to wash their genitalia and furniture which can easily be cleaned and decontaminated.

- Provide appropriate adult material, such as magazines or even DVDs.

Patients should be made to feel as relaxed and unhurried as possible, and staff at the sperm bank must do their utmost to ensure that the needs of the patient are prioritized over and above any time constraints of their own. If necessary, provisions should be made for staff to extend their hours in order to complete the process. Well-structured and comprehensible patient and service-user information (written and available online) can help to provide patients and their medical team with realistic expectations prior to their appointment. The extent to which the patient complies with the instructions given by the sperm bank will depend on a number of factors, including his age, level of comprehension, time constraints, and even level of motivation.

Although some men diagnosed with cancer may have poor semen quality prior to starting their treatment, current evidence would suggest that pretreatment semen quality is broadly similar across disease states (Bahadur et al., 2002) and is comparable with that of males without malignancies (Rofeim & Gilbert, 2004). However, it would be considered prudent to advise patients to provide multiple ejaculates wherever possible. The exact number of visits required and number of days' sexual abstinence between each will have to be assessed by senior sperm bank staff, although it has been shown that after taking into account postthaw quality an abstinence period between ejaculates of 24–48 hours is sufficient for most cancer patients (Agarwal et al., 1995).

Although it is well established that sperm motility and viability decreases significantly *after* cryopreservation and subsequent thawing (Agarwal et al., 2004), poor semen quality has not been shown to affect fertilization or pregnancy rates after cryopreservation and in vitro fertilization (IVF) or ICSI as long as live sperm can be recovered (see Chapter 8).

Unfortunately, a proportion of men or adolescents attending the sperm bank will be unable to provide an ejaculate by masturbation or use a condom to provide a sample by intercourse (if they have a partner). Anejaculation (AE) may result from neurological defects, such as spinal cord injury, and other relatively less common causes like multiple sclerosis, diabetes mellitus, or psychogenic or idiopathic causes. Penile vibratory stimulation (PVS), rectal probe electro-ejaculation (EEJ), and, as a last resort, surgical sperm retrieval (SSR) may be used obtain a specimen as outlined below.

Retrograde ejaculation

Retrograde ejaculation (RE) is classically caused by damage to the integrity of the bladder neck and posterior urethra (anatomical, trauma, neurogenic, drug-induced) leading to abnormal function of the internal sphincter of the urethra that favors ejaculation into the bladder (retrograde) as the path of least resistance (Aust & Lewis-Jones, 2004). Among patients attending an infertility clinic, RE is found most commonly in those with retroperitoneal lymph node dissection (RPLND), diabetes, posttraumatic paraplegia, after bladder-neck surgery, and treatment with either cytotoxic drugs (alkylating agents) or antidepressant and antipsychotic medication (haloperidol, thioridazine, fluxetin). However, often there is no obvious cause (idiopathic).

In cases of RE, sperm can be retrieved from the bladder after orgasm, but are usually nonviable and this precludes effective cryopreservation. Sperm entering the bladder are damaged because of the relative acidity and hypo-osmolarity of urine. Various protocols have been developed to raise the bladder pH and adjust the osmolarity by oral intake of sodium bicarbonate, but success has been variable (reviewed by Aust & Lewis-Jones, 2004). However, Aust et al. (2007) have systematically examined the physiology of urinary alkalinization and developed a protocol that leads to a urinary pH and osmolarity which can sustain sperm motility similar to that observed in culture media. However, its application to men with RE who are attempting to bank sperm remains to be proven. Although most men with RE will be able to urinate after ejaculation (and appropriate urinary alkalinization), in some, especially those with severe damage to the bladder neck and who also have problems with urinary incontinence, postejaculatory catheterization may be a more effective means to recover spermatozoa.

As an alternative to urinary alkalinization, other medical approaches can be attempted. For example, in men whose ejaculatory dysfunction is either neuropathic or associated with bladder neck scarring, sympathomimetic agents may enhance seminal emission and partially or completely convert the patient to antegrade ejaculation. Some standard regimens include pseudoephedrine hydrochloride 60 mg q.i.d, ephedrine sulfate 25–50 mg. q.i.d, phenylpropanolamine hydrochloride 75 mg b.i.d., and imipramine hydrochloride 25 mg q.i.d, Surgical reconstruction of the bladder neck has been attempted in the past, but it is not indicated today owing to advances in semen processing techniques. If all else fails, SSR may still be used to obtain viable sperm either from the testis or the epididymis (see later in this chapter).

Penile vibratory stimulation

For patients who are unsuccessful by either masturbation or by intercourse using a collection condom, Penile vibratory stimulation (PVS) is the first-line and least invasive available alternative. PVS is able to stimulate ejaculation in up to 80 percent of spinal cord injury cases and is useful in men (or adolescents) with psychogenic anejaculation. Patients with psychogenic anejaculation may be unwell, healthy adults, or adolescents who cannot consciously ejaculate by masturbation, although they may have erections and nocturnal emissions (Hovav et al., 2002). The medical PVS device is usually a simple handheld vibrator, which is applied to frenulum of the penis and has adjustable amplitude and frequency (Figure 6.4). To avoid unnecessary contamination and reduce biohazards risks, it is advisable that patients use this device in conjunction with the collection condom described earlier (Figure 6.3). Those using PVS because of spinal cord injury should do so with caution as men with injury above the T6 level are prone to a condition known as autonomic dysreflexia (AD), which results in a loss of control of blood pressure. Sperm banks should therefore ensure that communication with the referring department is effective and appropriate advice is sought from the spinal physician where indicated. AD can be controlled by appropriate administration of calcium channel-blockers such as nifedipine. The ejaculate obtained by PVS depends largely on the reason for AE. Sperm motility is often poor in spinal cord injury patients, owing to prolonged stasis during epididymal storage, but this may be normal in patients with psychogenic AE (Sønksen & Ohl, 2002). In either circumstance, sperm will be useable for some form of assisted conception (see Chapter 8).

Electro-ejaculation

When medical treatment for RE using sympathomimetics is unsuccessful in producing emission and ejaculation, electro-ejaculation (EEJ) has been shown to be an effective treatment option in over 70 percent of these patients (Ohl et al., 1991). Regardless of the reasons for anejaculation, ejaculates obtained with EEJ are often of poor quality, showing decreased concentration, motility, and viability (Brackett et al., 1994). When spermatozoa obtained by EEJ are used for intrauterine inseminations (IUI), the pregnancy rate per cycle

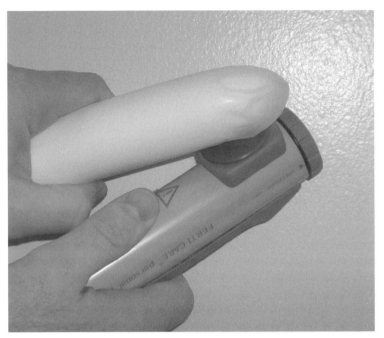

Figure 6.4 The FERTI CARE® personal penile vibrator for use in men with anejaculation. The picture illustrates how the vibratory pad is applied to the frenulum of the penis, illustrated in the picture by a condom-covered tube.

is 9–12 percent (Chung *et al.*, 1995; Ohl *et al.*, 2001). ICSI has resulted in improved fertility rates but with a median 60 percent fertilization rate, 15 percent pregnancy rate per cycle, and a 29 percent pregnancy rate per couple, these remain relatively poor (Schatte *et al.*, 2000). The low pregnancy rate achieved with sperm from these men is often attributed to low sperm motility, whose etiology may be related to detrimental effects of the electro-ejaculation process itself (Hovav *et al.*, 2002). The asthenozoospermia in spinal cord-injured patients may be related to increased scrotal temperature, urinary infection, stasis of seminal fluid, neural effects on physiology of the testis and epididymis, sperm auto-immunity, or external testicular pressure effects from the "closed-leg" position (Brackett *et al.*, 2000).

The semen quality resulting from PVS compared with EEJ is different. The more favorable results with PVS may be attributed to the fact that ejaculation by PVS is considered more physiological than by electro-ejaculation, and this is why PVS should be considered as a treatment of first choice. EEJ requires premedication (nifedipine) to prevent heart con-ductance defects with general anesthesia and thus may be used as a second-choice treatment, or indeed some fertility specialists may prefer to move straight to SSR, described below.

Surgical sperm retrieval

SSR is often the last option if all other attempts to collect sperm fail or, indeed, if the patient appears to be azoospermic after semen analysis. SSR is clearly an option open only to those patients who are deemed suitable, and it may be difficult to organize for those who require urgent cancer therapies. SSR is an "all-encompassing" term for a number of related tech-niques including: percutaneous epididymal sperm aspiration (PESA); testicular sperm aspiration (TESA); testicular sperm extraction (TESE); and microsurgical epididymal

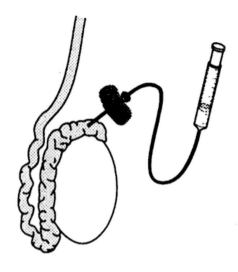

Figure 6.5 Diagrammatic representation of the percutaneous epididymal sperm aspiration (PESA) procedure. Reproduced by kind permission of Anthony Hirsch and redrawn from Hirsch (1997).

sperm aspiration (MESA). The choice of technique will largely be governed by the type of patient and his particular diagnosis, and some methods are a natural progression of others, depending the level of exploration required to find viable sperm.

PESA

PESA is the least invasive SSR technique and may easily be performed as an outpatient procedure. The patient requires conscious sedation and/or spermatic cord blockage with marcaine or lidocaine. The testis is immobilized with one hand while the aspiration is carried out with a butterfly needle (25-G) connected to a 20 cc plastic syringe, inserted through the scrotum directly into the proximal caput of the epididymis. A negative pressure is created by pulling the syringe plunger and epididymal fluid will be seen flowing into the plastic tubing of the butterfly needle (Figure 6.5). The fluid is then examined under the microscope in the laboratory to check for motile sperm and cryopreserved if necessary (see Chapter 7).

If no sperm are found, six to eight aspirates from each side should be carried out before switching to TESA or TESE, outlined below. The percentage of success (retrieval of motile spermatozoa) with PESA is about 93 percent (Ramos *et al.*, 2004). The advantages of PESA, in relation to MESA, are minimal discomfort for the patient and a lower complication rate, and it is also less expensive when compared with open surgery.

TESA and TESE

Testicular sperm retrieval involves either an open surgical biopsy or a percutaneous procedure. Sperm retrieval by open biopsy is termed "testicular sperm extraction" (TESE) and sperm retrieved percutaneously is termed "testicular sperm aspiration" (TESA) (Schlegel *et al.*, 1998).

Although a more invasive procedure, open surgical biopsy provides more tissue for harvesting sperm than does an aspiration procedure. TESA is generally sufficient for sperm retrieval from obstructed infertile men with normal spermatogenesis. It is an office procedure performed under local anesthesia. TESA uses transcutaneous aspiration by inserting a needle of 19–21 gauge directly into the testicular parenchyma and using negative pressure (Figure 6.6). The number of passes through the testicular tissue may vary from one to ten.

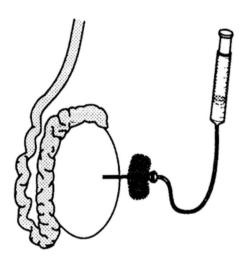

Figure 6.6 Diagrammatic representation of the testicular sperm aspiration (TESA) procedure. Reproduced by kind permission of Anthony Hirsch and redrawn from Hirsch (1997).

Retrieval of spermatozoa by TESA is less successful in the case of severely compromised spermatogenesis. In these instances, TESE should be the preferred method for harvesting spermatozoa.

For TESE, after spermatic cord anesthesia with marcaine 0.5 percent, a 1-cm transversal incision is carried through the scrotum and tunica vaginalis down to the tunica albuginea and tissue from the mid anterior surface of the testis is obtained. A single biopsy is generally sufficient for the ICSI procedure and for freezing any excess testicular spermatozoa. However, in some cases up to four biopsies (in different topographical sites) may be required (Tournaye et al., 1996).

There are many protocols to extract spermatozoa from the testicular tissue. Some (Bachtell et al., 1999) place the tissue at 37 °C in Earls medium (Gibco, Grand Island, NY) supplemented with 4.0 mmol/L of sodium bicarbonate (Fisher Scientific, Santa Clara, CA), 21 mmol/L HEPES (Calbiochem, La Jolla, CA), 0.47 mmol/L pyruvate (Sigma, St. Louis, MO), 100 U/mL penicillin, 50 µg/mL streptomycin sulfate, and 10 percent v/v synthetic serum substitute (Irvine Scientific, Santa Ana, CA) and then proceed with maceration to obtain testicular sperm. Others (DeCroo et al., 1998) place the homogenized testicular tissue in Earle medium at 37 °C supplemented with 0.1 percent of heparin and 0.4 percent of human serum albumin. Freezing is performed in much the same way as for ejaculated sperm.

Microscopic TESE has recently been used in conjunction with open biopsy and is conceptually similar to multibiopsy TESE, with several distinct differences: a single long testis incision is made to expose a large area of the testicular parenchyma and to access germ cell tubules, and a microscope is used for selecting the seminiferous tubules to be excised (Schlegel, 1999). The assumption is that the seminiferous tubules containing spermatogenic activity will appear more dilated (Bachtell et al., 1999) however this technique is much more invasive and requires general anaesthesia. Since the sperm that are obtained from the micro-TESE procedure are low in number and freeze very poorly, this procedure is generally performed the same day as egg retrieval during IVF, so as an option for the cancer patient wanting to bank sperm it may be of limited effectiveness. However, TESE will recover spermatozoa in approximately 40–45 percent of azoospermic patients who received chemotherapy for variety of cancers. TESE outcome is even higher in survivors of testicular cancer with persistent azoospermia after chemotherapy compared with other cancers causing azoospermia, with sperm retrieval rates of 67–75 percent (Chan et al., 2001; Mesenguer et al., 2003).

MESA

MESA combined with ICSI represented a great advance in the therapy of nonreconstructable obstructive azoospermia (Schroeder-Printzen et al., 2000). The procedure involves exposure of the epididymis through a c. 12 mm incision made in the scrotal skin. An operating microscope is used to identify and open the epididymal tubule to carry out the epididymal sperm aspiration. MESA is a successful technique to retrieve sperm from the epididymis in more than 90 percent of obstructive azoospermia cases (Silber et al., 1990; Collins et al., 1996; Oates et al, 1996; Holden et al., 1997; Patrizio, 2000). Lately, however, MESA is becoming an obsolete technique and has been replaced by the less invasive PESA method.

Sperm recovery in adolescents

Preserving the fertility of younger cancer patients requires coordinated efforts and attention to ethical issues by oncologists and fertility specialists (Robertson, 2005). Adequate counseling and support for adolescent cancer patients and their parents are essential prior to obtaining consent (see Chapter 4). Sperm cryopreservation in postpubertal adolescent patients may be performed with overall success rates similar to those observed in adults (Kamischke et al., 2004). It is possible to find sperm from ejaculated semen in boys aged 12 years and older, where the sperm are potentially useful for assisted reproductive techniques (Bahadur et al., 2002). In most cases a semen sample can be produced by masturbation, but if this is not possible, penile vibrostimulation or electro-ejaculation under anesthesia may be attempted (Muller et al., 2000; Grundy et al., 2001).

Cancer in children and options for fertility preservation

The incidence in the USA of childhood cancer is approximately 141 new cases per million annually, and leukemia is the most common childhood cancer, accounting for approximately 30 percent of cancers diagnosed in children aged less than 15 years (US Cancer Statistics Working Group, 2004). It is also estimated that one in 650 children are stricken by cancer and that 70–80 percent of them will survive. Of the survivors, about 20 percent will be permanently infertile (Jemal et al., 2004). If all germ line stem cells have been depleted after intense cancer therapy, no chances for spermatogenic recovery are available as yet. For prepubertal children, there are no current options available to preserve fertility, although a number of experimental approaches are being developed. These are discussed in more detail in Chapter 9.

Sperm retrieval after medical treatment

After gonadotoxic treatment, many men are obviously concerned about their fertility, and posttreatment semen analysis is recommended regardless of the type of therapy they have received. Data about posttreatment semen quality remain limited, although Bahadur et al. (2005) found that across all disease states only 37 percent of patients had posttreatment azoospermia after a mean follow-up period of 48.6 months. Similarly, Herr et al. (1998), who showed that over a 10-year follow-up period of men with stage 1 testis tumour that 65 percent of couples whom attempted a pregnancy were successful, and Brydøy et al. (2005) found that of 1814 men previously diagnosed with testicular cancer, the 15-year actuarial posttreatment paternity rate was 71 percent without the use of cryopreserved sperm. Clearly, following some treatments (e.g. total body irradiation) the rate of spontaneous pregnancy is known to be very low, although a handful of pregnancies has been reported (Pakkala *et al.*, 1994; Check *et al.*, 2000). Despite these apparent successes some post-treatment complications do exist and these are outlined below.

Post-cancer erectile and ejaculatory dysfunction

There are three major disorders of ejaculation: premature ejaculation; retrograde ejaculation; and ejaculatory failure. Retrograde ejaculation (RE) is the most common cause of ejaculatory dysfunction after pelvic radical surgery in cancer patients. Erectile dysfunction (ED) is the consistent inability to achieve or maintain an erection sufficient for satisfactory sexual performance (Kaye & Jick, 2003). Any surgical procedure that can harm or destroy nerve bundles controlling erection may result in ED, and about 50–80 percent of men who have a radical prostatectomy become impotent. Radiation therapy can damage arteries that provide blood flow to the penis, and may also cause scar tissue that may affect the dynamic of the erection. ED as a result of radiation therapy may not be as immediate as with surgery and may occur many months or even years after the treatment. The techniques used for sperm recovery in this situation include medical (e.g. one of the many phosphodiesterase inhibitors), surgical, and psychological therapy.

Posttreatment azoospermia

Gonadotoxic effects of cancer therapy on spermatogenesis are variable and patients can unpredictably become permanently azoospermic or severely or mildly oligozoospermic. It is estimated that at least 90 percent of young males become acutely azoospermic during cytotoxic therapy. Depending on type and dosage of the agent, resolution of azoospermia occurs in approximately 50 percent of these patients over a period of six month to five years (DeSantis *et al.*, 1999). Azoospermia can be caused by testicular failure (non-obstructive azoospermia) or it may be the result of a blockage of the male reproductive tract (obstructive azoospermia).

Non-obstructive azoospermia comprises the majority of cases in cancer patients and is a condition reflecting a severe spermatogenic compromise. The general histological patterns found in non-obstructive azoospermic patients are Sertoli cell only (in 60 percent, only Sertoli cells are present, with no germ cells in seminiferous tubules), maturation arrest (in 5 percent, Sertoli cells and immature germ cells are present in seminiferous tubules), and hypospermatogenesis (in 35 percent, there is a low number of germ cells and spermatids may or may not be present) (Tsujimura *et al.*, 2002). In obstructive azoospermia, although sperm production is maintained, sperm are trapped within the epididymis. Blockage may be caused directly by the tumor as a "mass effect" (i.e. prostate cancer, intratesticular cancer, and so on), or by the anticancer surgical therapy (i.e. retroperitoneal lymph-adenectomy) that could disrupt the normal anatomy and create an obstruction. Sperm harvesting techniques used to obtain sperm from men with obstructive and non-obstructive azoospermia include either testicular sperm retrieval (for men with non-obstructive azoospermia) or epididymal sperm aspiration (for men with obstructive azoospermia), as outlined earlier in this chapter. In the absence of any banked sperm, sperm recovered by these techniques may be used in assisted conception procedures (see Chapter 8).

Conclusion

Since the establishment of sperm banks the repertoire of techniques to obtain specimens for sperm banking has developed significantly, so that a variety of surgical and non-surgical procedures now exist to facilitate sperm storage. Although, at present, evidence suggests that only a minority of cancer patients will ever need to use their frozen samples in assisted conception procedures (see Chapter 8), all available opportunities should be explored at the outset to assist the cancer patient in banking sperm before the start of treatment.

References

Agarwal, A., Sidhu R.K., Shekarriz M. & Thomas A.J., Jr. (1995). Optimum abstinence time for cryopreservation of semen in cancer patients. *Journal of Urology*, **154**, 86–8.

Agarwal, A., Ranganathan, P., Kattal, N. *et al.* (2004). Fertility after cancer: a prospective review of assisted reproductive outcome with banked semen specimens. *Fertility and Sterility*, **81**, 342–8.

Aust, T.R. & Lewis-Jones, D.I. (2004). Retrograde ejaculation and male infertility. *Hospital Medicine*, **65**, 361–4.

Aust, T.R., Brookes, S., Troup, S.A., Fraser, W. D. & Lewis-Jones, D.I. (2007). Development and in vitro testing of a new method of urine preparation for retrograde ejaculation; the Liverpool solution. *Fertility and Sterility*, **89**, 885–91.

Bachtell, N.E., Conaghan, J. & Turek, P.J. (1999). The relative viability of human spermatozoa from the vas deferens, epididymis and testis before and after cryopreservation. *Human Reproduction*, **14**, 3048–51.

Bahadur, G., Ling, K.L., Hart, R. *et al.* (2002). Semen quality and cryopreservation in adolescent cancer patients. *Human Reproduction*, **17**, 3157–61.

Bahadur, G., Nahadur, G., Ozturk, O. *et al.* (2005). Semen quality before and after gonadotoxic treatment. *Human Reproduction*, **20**, 774–81.

Brackett, N.L., Lynne, C.M., Weizman, M.S., Bloch, W.E. & Abae, M. (1994). Endocrine profiles and semen quality of spinal cord injured men. *Journal of Urology*, **151**, 114–19.

Brackett, N.L., Lynne, C. M., Aballa, T.C. & Ferrell, S.M. (2000). Sperm motility from vas deferens of spinal cord injured men is higher than from ejaculate. *Journal of Urology*, **164**, 712–15.

Brougham, M.F., Kelnar, C.J., Sharpe, R.M. & Wallace, W.H. (2003). Male fertility following childhood cancer: current concepts and future therapies. *Asian Journal of Andrology*, **5**, 325–37.

Brydøy, M., Fosså, S.D., Klepp, O. *et al.* (2005). Paternity following treatment for testicular cancer. *Journal of the National Cancer Institute*, **97**, 1580–8.

Chan, P.T., Palermo, G.D., Veeck, L.L., Rosenwaks, Z. & Schlegel, P.N. (2001). Testicular sperm extraction combined with intracytoplasmic sperm injection in treatment of men with persistant azoospermia post chemotherapy. *Cancer*, **92**, 1632–7.

Check, M.L., Brown, T. & Check, J.H. (2000). Recovery of spermatogenesis and successful conception after bone marrow transplant for acute leukaemia: case report. *Human Reproduction*, **15**, 83–5.

Chung, P.H., Yeko, T.R., Mayer, J.C., Sanford, E. J. & Maroulis, G.B. (1995). Assisted fertility using electroejaculation in men with spinal cord injury. *Fertility and Sterility*, **64**, 1–9.

Collins, G.N., Critchlow, J.D., Lau, M.W.M. & Payne, S.R. (1996). Open versus closed epididymal sperm retrieval in men with secondarily obstructed vasal systems – a preliminary report. *British Journal of Urology*, **78**, 437–9.

DeCroo, I., Van der Elst, J., Everaert, K., De Sutter, P. & Dhont, M. (1998). Fertilization, pregnancy and embryo implantation rates after ICSI with fresh or frozen – thawed testicular spermatozoa. *Human Reproduction*, **13**, 1893–7.

DeSantis, M., Albrecht, W., Höltl, W. & Pont, J. (1999). Impact of cytotoxic treatment on long-term fertility in patients with germ-cell cancer. *International Journal of Cancer*, **83**, 864–5.

Grundy, R., Gosden, R.G., Hewitt, M. *et al.* (2001). Fertility preservation for children treated for cancer (1): scientific advances and research dilemmas. *Archives of Disease in Childhood*, **84**, 355–9.

Hallak, J., Kolettis, P.N., Sekhon, V.S., Thomas, A.J. Jr. & Agarwal, A. (1999). Sperm cryopreservation in patients with testicular cancer. *Urology*, **54**, 894–9.

Herr, H.W., Bar-Chama, N., O'Sullivan, M. & Sogani, P.C. (1998). Paternity in men with stage I testis tumors on surveillance. *Journal of Clinical Oncology*, **16**, 733–4.

Hirsch, A.V. (1997). A guide to the practice in andrology in the assisted conception unit. In P.A. Rainsbury & D.A. Viniker, eds., *Practical Guide to Reproductive Medicine*. Carnforth, UK: Parthenon Publishing.

Holden, C.A., Fuscaldo, G.F., Jackson, P. et al. (1997). Frozen–thawed epididymal spermatozoa for intracytoplasmatic sperm injection. *Fertility and Sterility*, **67**, 81–7.

Hovav, Y., Almagor, M. & Yaffe, H. (2002). Comparison of semen quality obtained by electroejaculation and spontaneous ejaculation in men suffering from ejaculation disorder. *Human Reproduction*, **17**, 3170–2.

Jemal, A., Clegg, L.X., Ward, E. et al. (2004). Annual report to the nation on the status of cancer, 1975–2001, with a specific feature regarding survival. *Cancer*, **101**, 3–27.

Kamischke, A., Jurgens, H., Hertle, L. et al. (2004). Cryopreservation of sperm from adolescents and adults with malignancies. *Journal of Andrology*, **25**, 586–92.

Kaye, J.A. & Jick, H. (2003). Incidence of erectile dysfunction and characteristics of patients before and after the introduction of sildenafil in the United Kingdom: cross-sectional study with comparison patients. *British Medical Journal*, **326**, 424–5.

Lass, A., Abusheikha, N., Akagbosu, F. & Brinsden, P. (1999). Cancer patients should be offered semen cryopreservation. *British Medical Journal*, **318**, 559–62.

Meistrich, M.L. (1999). Restoration of spermatogenesis by hormone treatment after cytotoxic therapy. *Acta Paediatrica* (Suppl.), **88**, 19–22.

Mesenguer, M., Garrido, N., Remohi, J. et al. (2003). Testicular sperm extraction (TESE) and ICSI in patients with permanent azoospermia after chemotherapy. *Human Reproduction*, **18**, 1281–5.

Muller, J., Sonksen, J., Sommer, P. et al. (2000). Cryopreservation of semen from pubertal boys with cancer. *Medical and Pediatric Oncology*, **34**, 191–4.

Oates, R.D., Lobel, S.M., Harris, D.H. et al. (1996). Efficacy of intracytoplasmatic sperm injection using intentionally cryopreserved epididymal spermatozoa. *Human Reproduction*, **11**, 133–8.

Ohl, D.A., Denil, J., Bennett, C.J. et al. (1991). Electroejaculation following retroperitoneal lymphadenectomy. *Journal of Urology*, **145**, 980–3.

Ohl, D.A., Wolf, L.J., Menge, A.C. et al. (2001). Electroejaculation and assisted reproductive technologies in the treatment of anejaculatory infertility. *Fertility and Sterility*, **76**, 1249–55.

Pakkala, S., Lukka, M., Helminen, P., Koskimies, S. & Ruutu, T. (1994). Paternity after bone marrow transplantation following conditioning with total body irradiation. *Bone Marrow Transplant*, **13**, 489–90.

Patrizio, P. (2000). Cryopreservation of epididymal sperm. *Molecular and Cellular Endocrinology*, **27**, 11–14.

Ramos, L., Wetzels, A.M., Hendriks, J.C. et al. (2004). Percutaneous epididymal sperm aspiration: a diagnostic tool for the prediction of complete spermatogenesis. *Reproductive Biomedicine Online*, **8**, 657–63.

Robertson, J.A. (2005). Cancer and fertility: ethical and legal challenges. *Journal of the National Cancer Institute Monographs*, **34**, 104–6.

Rofeim, O. & Gilbert, B.R. (2004) Normal semen parameters in cancer patients presenting for cryopreservation before gonadotoxic therapy. *Fertility and Sterility*. **82**, 505–6.

Schatte, E.C., Orejuela, F.J., Lipshultz, L.I., Kim, E.D. & Lamb, D.J. (2000). Treatment of infertility due to anejaculation in the male with electroejaculation and intracytoplaspic sperm injection. *Journal of Urology*, **163**, 1717–20.

Schlegel, P.N. (1999). Testicular sperm extraction; micro dissection improves sperm yield with minimal tissue excision. *Human Reproduction*, **14**, 131–5.

Schlegel, P.N., Su, L.M. & Li, P.S. (1998). Gonadal sperm retrieval: potential for testicular damage in non-obstructive azoospermia. In M. Fillicori & C. Flamigni, eds., *Treatment of Infertility: The New Frontiers*. New Jercy, NJ: Communications Media for Education, pp. 383–92.

Schover, L.R., Brey, K., Lichtin, A., Lipshultz, L.I. & Jeha, S. (2002). Knowledge and experience regarding cancer, infertility, and sperm banking in younger male survivors. *Journal of Clinical Oncology*, **20**, 1880–9.

Schroeder-Printzen, I., Zumbé, J., Bispink, L. et al. (2000). Microsurgical epididymal sperm aspiration: aspirate analysis and straws available after cryopreservation in patients with non-reconstructable obstructive azoospermia. *Human Reproduction*, **15**, 2531–5.

Shin, D., Lo, K.C. & Lipshultz, L.I. (2005). Treatment options for infertile male with cancer. *Journal of the National Cancer Institute Monographs*, **34**, 48–50.

Silber, S., Ord, T., Balmaceda, J., Patrizio, P. & Asch, R.H. (1990). Congenital absence of the vas deferens: studies on the fertilizing capacity of the human epididymal sperm. *New England Journal of Medicine*, **323**, 1788–92.

Sønksen J. & Ohl, D.A. (2002). Penile vibratory stimulation and electro-ejaculation in the treatment of ejaculatory dysfunction. *International Journal of Andrology*, **25**, 324–33.

Tournaye, H., Liu, J., Nagy, P.Z., Camus, M., Goossense, A., Silber, S., VanSteirteghem, A.C. & Devroey, P. (1996). Correlation between testicular histology and outcome after ICSI using testicular spermatozoa. *Human Reproduction*, **11**, 127–32.

Tsujimura, A., Matsumiya, K., Miyagawa, Y., *et al.* (2002). Conventional multiple or microdissection testicular sperm extraction: a comparative study. *Human Reproduction*, **17**, 2924–9.

US Cancer Statistics Working Group. (2004). *United Stated Cancer Statistics: 2000 Incidence and Mortality – Updated.* Atlanta, GA: Centers for Disease Control and Prevention and National Cancer Institute.

Sperm processing and storage

Mathew J. Tomlinson

Introduction

There are a number of important stages along the path to successful cryopreservation and, at each part of the process, technical and managerial weaknesses will adversely affect the final outcome (Figure 7.1). The purpose of this chapter is therefore to highlight the key requirements at each of these stages, from the initial semen quality evaluation and processing through to freezing and eventual storage in liquid nitrogen or nitrogen vapor. Suggestions for good practice are given and the need for careful management is emphasized, including validation of method, risk analysis, and quality assurance.

Semen analysis

Before samples are to be analyzed and processed prior to storage, they must be produced in satisfactory conditions. For diagnostic purposes, acceptance criteria for ejaculated specimens require that the analysis begins within an hour of its production after at least two days of sexual abstinence (WHO, 1999). However, with regard to patients facing life-saving cytotoxic therapy, to adhere to such standards may be optimistic. First, the need for the oncologist to commence therapy may well override the need to collect an optimal sample. In addition, sperm banks may not be as accessible as the local diagnostic laboratory and patients may feel uncomfortable at the prospect of producing the sample "on site." Sperm banks therefore tend to adopt a more flexible and relaxed approach toward their own specimen acceptance criteria and acknowledge that any sample is better than none if it is to be an individual's only prospect of future fatherhood. On delivery it is essential that the patient's identity is confirmed and that, for any specimen sent via a relative or courier, a clear and documented third-party "chain of custody" is in evidence. Equally important is that the sperm bank emphasizes the need for traceability and quality with regard to products that come into contact with the specimen, such as requiring the use of specimen containers provided by the clinic that have been tested previously for sperm toxicity. If time permits it may be an advantage for the patient to bank further samples, the number of which should be based on the considered opinion of senior sperm bank staff, taking into account his diagnosis and the relative quality of the samples already banked.

From a quality assurance perspective, it is imperative that semen analysis is only carried out using techniques which carry some clinical validation and that parameters are measured with the same care and accuracy as for diagnostic testing (WHO, 1999). Either a portion of sample should be removed for analysis (using a sterile pipette) or sterile pipette tips should be used throughout to avoid contamination prior to freezing. Sample processing within a laminar flow or class II cabinet to reduce the risk of microbial or particulate contamination

Sperm Banking: Theory and Practice, eds. Allan A. Pacey and Mathew J. Tomlinson.
Published by Cambridge University Press. © Cambridge University Press 2009.

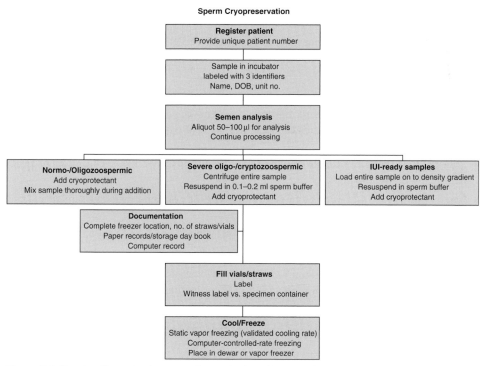

Figure 7.1 Flowchart illustrating the stages of sperm banking, from attendance at the laboratory to freezing of any sample provided.

is a sensible precaution and indeed is now obligatory among European Union (EU) member states since the adoption of the EU directive for cells and tissues in 2007. Grade A air (<1 cfu, <3.5 particles per m³) is now the EU standard processing environment for any sample (HFEA, 2007), coupled with a suitable (Grade D) background environment.

Sperm processing

Common practice in many sperm banks, is to store masturbatory ejaculates in their raw state (i.e. in seminal fluid). However, some commercial sperm banks, in particular in the USA, prepare donor sperm using density gradient centrifugation in order to produce an "insemination-ready" product. Some have demonstrated clear superiority by use of this method in terms of postthaw outcome (Sharma & Agarwal, 1997; Esteves *et al.*, 2000). The freezing of washed–prepared sperm units may have a number of other distinct advantages for the freezing and storage of sperm samples for men banking sperm for their own use. From a risk reduction perspective, the removal of any contaminating pathogens within the seminal fluid by simple gradient preparation is a sure way of reducing the likelihood of a cross-infection incident within a freezer. Evidence from clinics treating HIV-discordant couples (male positive, female negative) show that seminal viral load is reduced to almost undetectable levels by use of such methods (Kim *et al.*, 1999; Nicopoullos *et al.*, 2004). It is clearly desirable to store as "clean" a sample as is possible, particularly as some packaging materials are known to be less than perfect with regard to their integrity at liquid nitrogen temperatures (see later in this chapter). Moreover, the storage of smaller, more concentrated, sperm pellets, which use less freezer space and are of higher quality is an attractive one, especially for the patient with poorer quality sperm and for reducing the workload when treating patients with frozen samples at a later date (see Chapter 8).

Cryopreservative

There is little consensus over which cryopreservative or cryoprotectant medium is best (in terms of percentage yield of motile sperm postthaw), particularly as there are so many confounding variables which make comparative evaluation extremely difficult. These include whether:

- The methods used to evaluate outcome (sperm motility, viability, fertilization or pregnancy) are comparable.
- Sperm motility is measured manually or by use of computer-assisted semen analysis (CASA), and at room temperature or at 37 °C.
- The cooling rate used to freeze samples is constant for every sample.
- Cryoprotectant is added at exactly the same rate for every sample.
- The laboratory is capable of accurately evaluating sperm quality in the first place, given the known laboratory-to-laboratory variation in evaluating semen quality (Matson, 1995).

Early cryoprotectants were home-made and based around the use of glycerol and egg yolk (McLaughlin *et al.*, 1992). However, recent anxiety about the use of animal products in media intended for human use have led to concern over their use (Alvarez & Storey, 1993; Tomlinson, 2005). Many sperm banks are therefore turning toward one of the many commercially licensed products now available (which are generally free of egg yolk, although many are still supplemented with a human serum albumin). These have proven efficacy, batch-to-batch consistency, are easily validated, and include products such as Sperm Freeze (Fertipro, Belgium), Sperm Freezing Medium (MediCult UK), and Sperm Cryoprotec™ (Nidacon, Sweden) among others.

Penetrating cryoprotectants based on glycerol promote cell dehydration, minimizing the deleterious effect of inappropriate ice crystal formation as well as restricting toxic solution effects. Cryopreservation without them will result in an unacceptable outcome in terms of postthaw motility, membrane integrity, and cell viability (see Chapter 1). Cryoprotectants should be added slowly enough to allow permeation to reach equilibrium (avoiding osmotic shock) but balanced carefully against the need to avoid glycerol toxicity (McLaughlin *et al.*, 1992). Most commercial providers of cryoprotectant advocate the drop-by-drop addition of cryoprotectant, but without specifying either the size of the drop or the rate of addition. Gao and co-workers (1995) showed that a four-step addition of a fixed molarity (1 M) of glyercol with only 1–2 minutes between each two steps achieved satisfactory osmotic equilibration, minimizing toxicity and significantly reducing deterioration in motility and viability. This had to be coupled with an eight-step removal process (addition of washing buffer) during thaw; again, to minimize osmotic damage to sperm membranes.

The containment (packaging) system

The containment system used to store a patient's sperm is all-important. To be perfectly effective, it must satisfy a number of important criteria.

- Provide a large surface area:volume ratio to maximize heat exchange and allow uniform cooling of the sample.

- Available in small, easy to use units that may be thawed for treatment without wastage.
- Available in sterilized units.
- Form an impenetrable seal even when immersed in liquid nitrogen.
- Able to withstand ultra-low temperatures without breakage.
- Provide space for clear labeling.
- Easy to manipulate and recognize (e.g. during audit or removal for later use).

Obviously, packaging materials used in other clinical areas to freeze patient material (e.g. blood bags) would be totally inappropriate for banking sperm. For human sperm storage there are few options. Traditionally, clinics have stored in 0.25–0.5 mL straws or paillettes (IMV, France). These were developed for the veterinary industry and were originally made from polyvinyl chloride (PVC) and are now made from polyterepthalate glycol (PTEG) (Mortimer, 2004). Over the years these have been widely used, and they certainly satisfy most of the criteria mentioned above. Their considerable advantage lies in providing even heat exchange throughout the sample and hence uniform cooling. The excellent review by Mortimer (2004) describes how, of the packaging systems available, only straws provide an environment for optimum cooling of sperm, particularly when compared with that provided by plastic cryovials (Figure 7.2).

Data from our own laboratory have shown clearly that the cooling rate of samples frozen in the center of a cryovial is least 1 °C slower than the sample adjacent to the inner vial wall. In terms of convenience and providing small units for use in treatment, PVC/PTEG straws are more than adequate, although their integrity at ultra-low temperatures and the effectiveness of the polyvinyl alcohol (PVA) powder seal has certainly come into question. Like many materials, they become very fragile after long-term immersion in liquid nitrogen and may break very easily. The sealing method, which involves tamping down onto PVA powder to form a plug, followed by "curing" (polymerization) in water is also a documented area of weakness (Clarke, 1999; Mortimer, 2004). A poor plug or insufficient "air-space" within the straw to allow for expansion during warming will lead to propulsion of the plug at high velocity (another reason to wear safety goggles in the cryo-room). An alternative sealing method is available with the CBS (Cryobiosystem) "high security straw" (CBS, France). These are made from an ionomeric resin, and have the same advantages as conventional straws in terms of heat exchange but, in addition, are very strong even at ultra-low temperatures and may be securely sealed by use of a thermal welding device known as the "Symms sealer." The combination of the strength of the CBS straw and its improved sealing method provides the best available bio-containment for human cells and tissues in liquid nitrogen storage. Figure 7.3 shows the filling, sealing and labeling sequence for the CBS straw system.

Cryovials such as those produced by Nunc (Nalgene International, Rochester, USA) have also been extensively used for storing sperm, particularly since the mid 1990s. The use of vials has been popularized by commercial sperm banks where convenience and the requirement for a single-dose treatment unit has possibly overridden the need for the optimum packaging system in terms of postthaw sperm yield. They are certainly easy to use, with filling and labeling being easier than with straws; yet, with relatively large diameters and semen volumes, uniform cooling of the sample is almost impossible to achieve. Moreover, laboratories still insist on storing cryovials in the liquid phase of nitrogen, a practice that is both hazardous and contrary to manufacturer's recommendation (Nunc, 2003). During cooling the vial is subject to significant shrinkage and embrittlement, and the contents

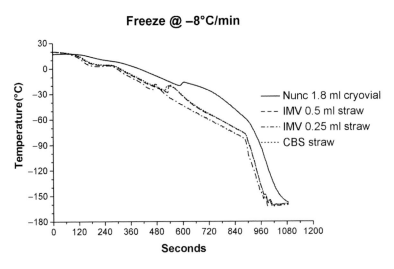

Freeze @ −8°C/min

Temperature(°C) vs Seconds

— Nunc 1.8 ml cryovial
--- IMV 0.5 ml straw
--·· IMV 0.25 ml straw
···· CBS straw

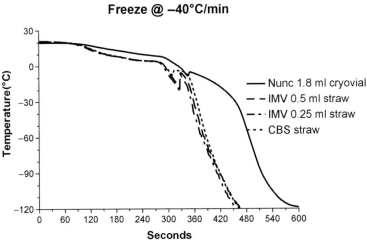

Freeze @ −40°C/min

Temperature(°C) vs Seconds

— Nunc 1.8 ml cryovial
-- IMV 0.5 ml straw
-·- IMV 0.25 ml straw
·· CBS straw

Figure 7.2 Cooling curves for straws versus vials showing more uniform cooling with straws. This figure is based on the unpublished data of Agnès Camus (CryoBioSystem, Paris, France). Reproduced from Mortimer (2004) with permission.

contract creating a vacuum which freely permits liquid nitrogen to be drawn into the vial. Upon thawing, liquid nitrogen expands to 700 times its original volume and, with no relief, the vial will explode. A survey conducted at the UK Association of Clinical Embryologists (ACE) joint annual meeting with the Irish Association of Embryologists (ICE) showed that a remarkably high proportion of embryologists had observed an exploding cryovial (Tomlinson & Morroll, 2008), injuries from which are well documented. Moreover, what if this trapped liquid nitrogen contains viral particles with the infectivity of Hepatitis B? There are clearly issues with cryovials in liquid nitrogen and thus their use should be limited to vapor-phase storage only.

Table 7.1 summarizes the advantages and disadvantages of the packing systems available, with regard to the essential criteria stated above. Based on this, the ionomeric resin straw would appear to be the only inventory option that satisfies all the necessary conditions for storage and is associated with the least risk. We should bear in mind, however, that

Table 7.1 *Advantages and disadvantages of various packaging for freezing sperm*

	Cryovials	PVC straws	PTEG straws	0.5 mL CBS straws
Uniform cooling – for optimum yields	✔	✔ ✔ ✔	✔ ✔ ✔	✔ ✔ ✔
Available in small, convenient units	✔ ✔ ✔	✔ ✔ ✔	✔ ✔ ✔	✔ ✔ ✔
Conveniently and effectively sealed	✔	✔	✔	✔ ✔ ✔
Robust at −196°C	✔ ✔ ✔	✔	✔	✔ ✔ ✔
Suitable for immersion in liquid nitrogen	✔	✔ ✔	✔ ✔	✔ ✔ ✔
Easy to label clearly	✔ ✔ ✔	✔	✔	✔ ✔
Easily manipulated and recognized, e.g. during audit	✔ ✔ ✔	✔	✔	✔ ✔

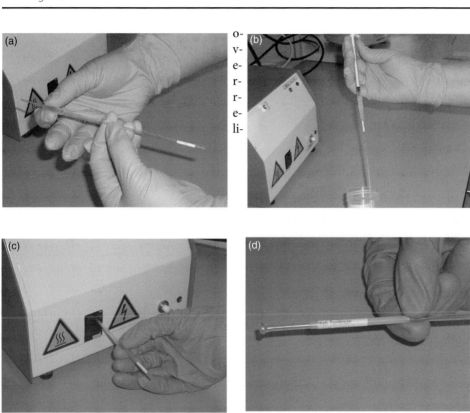

Figure 7.3 Filling and sealing procedure for CBS high-security straws: (a) fitting the sterile filling nozzle; (b) loading the straw with sperm or cryoprotectant mixture using a syringe; (c) sealing the straw ends using the Symms sealer; (d) the final sealed and labeled straw prior to cooling.

ance on any one system to solve biocontainment issues would be foolhardy, and a comprehensive risk management approach should implemented. Since the now infamous cross-contamination incident (Tedder *et al.*, 1995), in which patients were infected with Hepatitis B and the source of infection was traced to a burst blood bag stored in a liquid nitrogen vessel, general awareness of the issues surrounding risk and biocontainment are understandably heightened.

Labeling and handling

An important consideration when designing any inventory item is the quality of labeling and the ease with which individual units may be labeled, manipulated, and recognized. There are anecdotal reports of poor practice such as paper tags for labeling straws (these easily become detached during nitrogen immersion) and inaccurate and misaligned markings on straws (see below), which easily lead to misidentification. During an audit, handling straws for an inappropriately long period while attempting to read an unclear label could easily result in partial thaw and probably deterioration of sperm quality. Straws, in particular the 0.25 mL size, are particularly difficult to label, and many laboratories favor the French marking system: a three- or four-digit number that is represented on the straw by lines: one line for the first digit, two lines for the second digit, and so on. Great care must be taken in marking this way, as misalignment of the markings is very easy. Reading them during an audit is also particularly difficult, and overhandling to remove frost should be avoided. Cryovials are relatively easy to label and have a large enough space to write on with a cryopen. Centers are gradually moving toward automated labeling, either with label or bar-code printers in order to lessen the risk of transcription errors. The 0.5 mL CBS straws may be fitted with an external sleeve around which a printed label can be attached, as shown earlier in Figure 7.3(d).

Freezing

In comparison with embryo freezing, the cryopreservation of sperm is relatively crude. The majority of sperm banks still freeze sperm by a method first introduced by Sherman (1973), which involves suspending samples in nitrogen vapor for a period of time before plunging them into liquid nitrogen. Whether controlled-rate freezing (CRF) provides better results in terms of postthaw motility is a matter for debate. Computer-controlled freezers provide advantages above the manual methods related to validation and consistency, and they tend to work in one of two ways: first, by circulating nitrogen vapor in a controlled manner across samples lying within a dry chamber, as in the range of freezers by Planer (www. planer.co.uk): second, more recent "solid-state" designs in which samples are placed in a heated chamber which is placed directly in a liquid nitrogen reservoir, such as the Cryologic CL-8800r (www.cryologic.com) or the Biotronics DB-1 Embryofreeze (www.biotronics. net). Both methods appear to be effective, although the latter are becoming increasingly favored within the in vitro fertilization (IVF) laboratory owing to their compact design and the advantage of having no moving solenoid valves, pumps, or motors which may freeze or jam. A more recent development is the mechanical Grant Asymptote freezer (www.grant. co.uk), which does not use nitrogen as a coolant source but instead employs technology in the form of a Stirling engine. This "Stirling Cycle Cryocooler," as it is called, has been developed as an alternative to conventional liquid nitrogen controlled-rate freezers and is thought to pose a lower contamination risk, has a very compact design, and is relatively quiet in operation; this is thought to make it particularly suited to a clean-room environment. Early data suggest that this alternative has a number of applications in cryopreservation (Morris et al., 2006); however, a lengthy track record of successful freezing is what most sperm banks would prefer to see before making any radical changes in their approach.

Controlled-rate freezers typically have an inbuilt program for sperm freezing or they may be tailored to the needs of the sperm bank either by using a keypad or a PC link. Most sperm-freezing programs are designed to cool at an average of $-10\,°C$ per minute before

Table 7.2 *Concentration, motility, and velocity in 50 samples cooled using vapor freezing (VF) and a controlled-rate freezer (Planar protocol)*

Cooling method	VF (mean, min–max)	CRF (mean, min–max)
Concentration ($\times 10^6$/mL)	29.9	30.4
	(2.9–112)	(2.8–124)
Progressive motility (%)	9.1	8.6
	(1.1–41.2)	(1.1–56)
Progressive velocity (μm/s)	13.5	12.4
	(5.8–33.5)	(4.8–26.4)

plunging in nitrogen. However, some of the more recent compact freezers described above appear to struggle to achieve such a rapid cooling rate. A typical freezing program for sperm (adapted from Morris *et al.*, 1999) is shown below:

1. Start at 24°C (approximately room temperature).

2. Cooling rate 2°C per minute to −5°C

3. Cool at 10°C per minute from −5°C to −100°C.

4. Transfer to liquid (−196°C) or vapor phase (between approximately −150°C and −190°C) storage.

Users should be aware, however, that established cooling rates often relate to chamber temperatures and not the temperature of the sample, which may vary according to the packaging used. Therefore, in-house validation of specimen cooling rates requires the placing of thermocouples into cooling cryoprotectant before settling on a particular program. A study by Ragni and coworkers (1990) suggested that the use of controlled-rate freezers leads to better survival of poor samples (e.g. from oncology patients); this has been contradicted by others (Paras *et al.*, 2007). Straw-to-straw or vial-to-vial variation is more common when using conventional freezing methods, and this may not be a concern with donor sperm or those with normal semen parameters, but may be of more significance when freezing sperm of poorer quality such as that of the chronically ill patient. Using either the cooling program above, or a straight −10°C/minute rate, our laboratory found little difference between controlled-rate freezers and vapor freezing in terms of postthaw semen quality (Table 7.2). Equivalent survival rates with simple vapor cooling are therefore achievable providing the cooling rate is first carefully manipulated by adjusting the height or distance from the coolant source in order to provide the same rate as the controlled-rate freezer.

A number of alternative simple vapor freezing methods have been cited in the literature (Table 7.3). The fact that they provide dissimilar cooling curves yet are thought to be successful illustrates the relatively large tolerance of sperm to variations in cooling rates (see Chapter 1).

Whichever method is employed, documentation to support the cooling rate, and ultimately satisfactory evidence showing successful outcome in terms of postthaw sperm yield and pregnancies, should be basic quality assurance requirements within an accredited laboratory. The modern sperm bank ought to optimize its own system, considering a number of factors along with the type of cryoprotectant employed and not take for granted that a system that may work extremely well with 0.25 mL for straws is necessarily effective for cryovials.

Table 7.3 *Simple static vapor cooling procedures cited in the literature*

Suggested cooling procedure	Reference
1 hour @ 4 °C, followed by 15 minutes @ 37.5 cm above LN_2, followed by a further 15 minutes @ 27.5 cm	Saritha & Bongso (2001)
10 minutes @ 25 cm above LN_2 (for 0.25 mL straws)	Mortimer (2004)
15 minutes @ 10 cm above LN_2	Donnelly *et al.* (2001)
15 minutes @ 10 cm above the neck of a dry shipper, followed by 30 minutes at the bottom	Tomlinson & Barratt (2004)

Inventory design: storage racking

The design of the freezer furniture (or racking) is largely governed by the packaging system used, the size of vessel in use, and – to a degree – whether storage is carried out in the liquid or vapor phase of nitrogen. It must fulfill some basic needs with regard to minimizing sample losses: keeping them at an appropriate temperature (in particular during vapor storage) and permitting easy access to individual sample units. Sperm banks using straws tend to store them in individual freezing goblets stacked in a circular canister. In a standard medium-sized liquid dewar (e.g. Taylor Wharton 35HC) these will be stacked two deep (Figure 7.4).

If storing these in a large vapor refrigerator (e.g. Taylor Wharton 10K), these may be stacked up to four deep (Figure 7.5), in which case metal dividers could be inserted into each goblet to improve conductance and keep samples at the top of the inventory at similar temperatures to those at the bottom.

Storage in the vapor phase allows the use of perhaps more sophisticated racking designs, such as the large towers with individual drawers for cryovials. Alternatively, a simple canister system may be employed, which is particularly useful if, as in some older sperm banks, there is a mixture of straws and vials. In this case straws may be placed in goblets within visotubes and stacked toward the lower end of the freezer where it is colder. Vials clipped onto aluminium canes will improve thermal conductivity and help the freezer achieve very low temperatures toward the top of the inventory and may therefore be placed above the straws within the freezer (Figure 7.5). Plastic inventory or racking has been used by some manufacturers, but is wholly unsuitable for low-temperature storage in the vapor phase, as it overinsulates the samples furthest away from the nitrogen reservoir. When plastic canisters were used during testing of our own system, temperatures lower than −100 °C could not be achieved at the top of the inventory, which is clearly some distance from the critical −130 °C to −140 °C range required for long-term storage. In vapor, packing the freezer both with samples and with as much highly conductive material as possible is essential to ensure temperature stabilization. Aluminium or steel containers should be used to house the samples and to improve conduction further; either cryocanes (often used with cryovials) or aluminium canister or goblet dividers may also be used to lower the temperature and provide a necessary safety margin. Any significant gaps between inventory towers or canisters may be filled with lengths of metal such as copper pipe, to improve freezer efficiency further. The large towers with drawers for cryovials provide suitable conductivity but do not permit the easy storage of different containment systems (i.e. they are limited to vials). Moreover, access to the bottom drawer requires the removal of the entire tower, which is bulky and cumbersome, and not recommended if the freezer contents

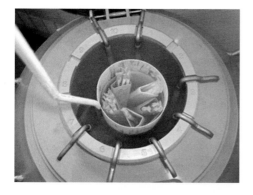

Figure 7.4 Frozen straws held in triangular visitubes and contained within a goblet for storage within a medium-sized liquid nitrogen dewar (e.g. Taylor Wharton 35HC).

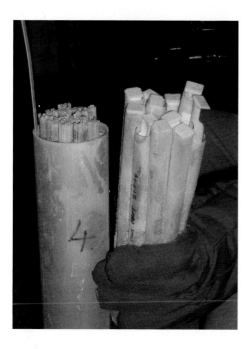

Figure 7.5 Long aluminium canisters for storage of a mixed inventory of straws and vials in a bulk refrigerator.

are to be accessed on a regular basis. A relatively full freezer, with an appropriately designed racking and inventory, will achieve temperatures as low as $-190°C$ just below the freezer lid with a temperature range of between $-175°C$ and $-190°C$ lower down (Tomlinson, 2005).

Long-term storage: liquid nitrogen or vapor phase

The long-term storage of living cells must take place at temperatures lower than approximately $-135°C$, the so-called "glassy transformation temperature" (Meryman, 1963). Although sperm may be successfully stored at higher temperatures in the short term (some commercial sperm donor banks transport samples on dry ice at $-79°C$), it has been shown that storage for long periods above $-135°C$ results in a progressive decline in postthaw sperm quality (Ackerman, 1968; Behrman & Ackerman, 1969). Storage in liquid nitrogen (liquid at $-196°C$) is preferable and has been used to freeze and store human

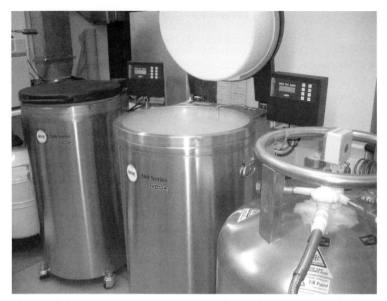

Figure 7.6 Bulk vapor storage freezers automatically supplied with nitrogen from a pressurized vessel.

sperm since the early 1970s (Smith & Steinberger, 1973; Barkey et al., 1974). The majority of laboratories storing sperm or embryos, or both, have tended to do so in medium-sized liquid nitrogen vessels (see Figure 7.4). Some larger sperm banks, however, in particular those storing samples for a large number of cancer patients, have reached a size that warrants the use of bulk refrigerators, which may be used for either liquid or vapor phase storage (Figure 7.6).

The drive toward storage in nitrogen vapor in the UK has been largely the result of the unfortunate incident mentioned previously, in which six patients contracted hepatitis from autologous transplant of their own blood stem cells stored in liquid nitrogen (Tedder et al., 1995). A broken blood bag from one patient who was Hepatitis B positive appeared to have led to the transmission of the virus to the other patients via the circulating liquid nitrogen. After this incident, the UK Department of Health (DoH) responded by proposing the following strategy for all long-term storage of blood products.

- Patients having cells stored should be screened for Hepatitis B and C, and for HIV1 and 2.
- Samples should have secondary sealed packaging.
- Samples should be stored in nitrogen vapor as a "safer" alternative.

As a consequence, both the UK National Blood Service and accredited tissue banks have now moved over to storage in the vapor phase (NHS Executive, 1997). Some laboratories even store human cells long term in mechanical −140°C freezers. Not without good reason has there been some reluctance by sperm banks in the UK to move toward storage in the vapor phase. There are concerns with the cost of the initial outlay and installation, concerns about whether suitable storage temperatures can be achieved, and certainly concern that there is little physical proof that vapor storage is inherently safer. These are all important considerations and the only sensible answer is that a move toward bulk storage should depend on the size of the facility and the quantity of storage being undertaken. Any unit wishing to store upwards of 5000 cryovials or 20 000 straws at any one time would find little difference in cost between purchasing a small vapor refrigerator, such as the Taylor Wharton 10K, and enough alarmed nitrogen dewars with a similar capacity. The major difference would be in the running costs: vapor freezers require more servicing and use on average four times the quantity of liquid nitrogen. In terms of achieving optimum storage temperature, there is no real difference between liquid- and vapor-phase storage. It is certainly the case that in nitrogen liquid the temperature will remain a stable at $-196\,°C$ and that in vapor this will fluctuate between approximately $-170\,°C$ and $-190\,°C$, depending on inventory design and sample numbers (Tomlinson, 2005). Yet, since biological activity ceases beyond $-135\,°C$, nothing is gained by cooling samples any further. If anything, all that is provided is an extra safety margin.

The advantage of the liquid nitrogen dewar is its simplicity. It is a very rudimentary piece of equipment with no moving parts, requiring little or no servicing, and is associated with a remarkably low failure rate. Because samples are constantly immersed in liquid nitrogen, it ensures that they will be maintained at a suitable (and constant) temperature. Adaptation of existing liquid nitrogen dewars, as suggested by Clarke (1999), is an alternative solution to storage in vapor, without the need for large-scale investment. However, vapor storage done in this way requires more elaborate monitoring and, although satisfactory temperatures may be obtained in a dewar with only a few centimeters of nitrogen in the bottom, there are obvious implications for dewar capacity as the lower layer of the dewar is used as the nitrogen reservoir. For the average-sized dewar, this leaves enough canister height for only a single layer of straws and insufficient height for standard cryocanes. Furthermore, there is little point in keeping the inventory free from immersion in liquid in storage, filling the dewar from the top, given that liquid nitrogen has been shown to be a potential source of contamination (Fountain et al., 1997). Therefore, filling hoses have to be placed in the dewar bottom and the nitrogen level should be carefully checked until it reaches the desired level. The dewar will stay sufficiently cold even with 1–2 cm nitrogen in the bottom, but will warm rapidly once this evaporates (Tomlinson, 2005). Careful temperature and liquid level monitoring is required to reduce the risk of temperature fluctuations

The monitoring required by an automated vapor storage system (in comparison with liquid storage) is considerable, and relates to the scale of reliance on inherently risky autofilling systems. Faulty liquid level sensing may lead to failure to fill, or overfilling. Overfilling, in which the freezer fails to detect the maximum permitted liquid level and continues to fill, bathes the entire inventory in liquid nitrogen. This may not lead to sample losses but it is nevertheless extremely hazardous. First, it defeats the object of having vapor storage in the first place: without an extremely robust and leak-free containment system it may lead to the very cross-contamination incidents that vapor storage are designed to avoid. Second, overfilling may cause severe problems in the cryoroom leading to the complete emptying of the supply vessel; liquid will spill onto the floor, displace oxygen from the room, and reduce or completely interrupt the supply to other vessels. It was a faulty pressure sensor on a CBS isothermal unit vessel that led the UK Medicines and Healthcare Regulation Agency (www.mhra.gov.uk) to issue a general alert, recognizing for the first time that these vessels should perhaps be classed as medical devices. It is perhaps surprising that they had not done so previously, given the potential cost of loss of the cells and tissue being stored within them. Therefore, although an autofill system may seem quite an attractive function, laboratories must be aware of the potential pitfalls and ensure that the entire system is carefully planned and designed by expert engineers, and incorporates a number of inbuilt fail-safe features.

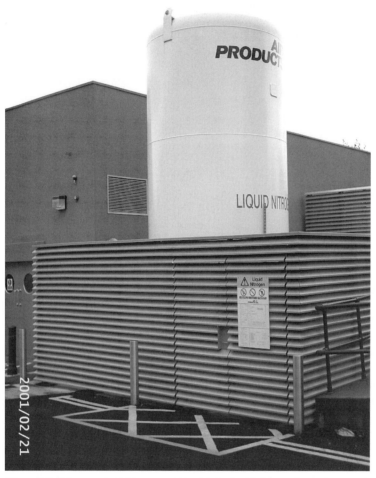

Figure 7.7 Bulk-pressurized storage vessel containing liquid nitrogen for use in sperm banks with a large capacity.

Ensuring a continuous nitrogen supply

The key to running an efficient sperm bank, especially one that is based on automated nitrogen vapor refrigeration, lies in ensuring that the nitrogen supply is maintained. Liquid vessels with small necks and low evaporation may be left for two to three weeks between fillings (although this is not considered best practice), but large vapor storage units with large-diameter lids suffer from relatively large liquid usage. Despite manufacturer's claims from test units, even small vapor freezers full of samples will use in excess of 20l of nitrogen per day (Tomlinson, personal observation). If multiple units are in use, then careful thought must be given to the liquid supply. As few as four units, using between 80l and 100l of nitrogen per day, would warrant the use of a large external bulk supply tank (Figure 7.7), otherwise staff would be changing supply vessels three or four times a week, which has significant health and safety implications given the risk of exposure to liquid nitrogen.

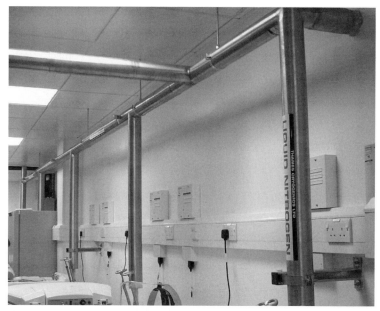

Figure 7.8 Super-insulated, vacuum-lined piping (SIVL) for the supply of vapor storage freezers (see Figure 7.6) from an external bulk-pressurized storage vessel (see Figure 7.7).

The bulk storage of nitrogen on-site would also help as a fail-safe in the event that the gas supplier failed to deliver. To minimize further losses, (super-insulated, vacuum-lined piping) (SIVL) is likely to be necessary and is now commonplace in large blood products storage or tissue storage facilities (Figure 7.8). Installation of vacuum-lined pipelines is expensive but the liquid nitrogen can remain within the line, significantly reducing losses and recovering initial outlay costs within a few years. Careful thought has to be given to the length of pipeline, relative to the freezer-filling interval. Too long a pipe run with a relatively large filling interval may require a substantial pipe-cooling phase, consuming large amounts of liquid nitrogen in the process. Ideally, the storage facility should be located on a ground floor with easy access for delivery and keeping pipe-run length to a minimum.

Table 7.4 shows the relative strengths and weaknesses of different types of equipment used in the long-term storage of sperm. On balance, storage in vapor appears to have a slight advantage, if only from a health and safety perspective, but clearly its use depends on the size of the service. Storage at −80 °C in a mechanical freezer is not sustainable without significant deterioration in sample quality. At −140 °C it may be more attractive although there is little margin for error in terms of temperature, the freezers are expensive, and dependent on a continuous power supply. If the perfect packaging system existed, with zero risk of breakage and a 100 percent effective seal, there would be little to choose between liquid- or vapor-phase nitrogen storage. We may even be close to this, but there is always unforeseeable human or mechanical error. For example, it would only take a faulty straw, sealing machine, or poorly trained technician to produce a defectively sealed unit and, consequently, potentially contaminate an entire storage vessel. The fail-safe in this case would be to keep samples in the most robust packaging system available but in nitrogen vapor.

Table 7.4 *Advantages and disadvantages of sperm storage equipment*

	Liquid nitrogen vessel	Automated nitrogen vapor vessel	Liquid vessel converted to vapor	−140°C mechanical freezer
Permits long-term storage < −135°C.	✔ ✔ ✔	✔ ✔ ✔	✔ ✔ ✔	✔ ✔
Safe for the operator and easily accessible	✔ ✔	✔ ✔ ✔	✔ ✔ ✔	✔ ✔ ✔
Low cost (purchase and running)	✔ ✔ ✔	✔	✔ ✔	N/A
Reduced risk of cross-infection	✔	✔ ✔ ✔	✔ ✔ ✔	✔ ✔ ✔
Integral data logging and alarm	✔	✔ ✔ ✔	✔	✔ ✔ ✔
High capacity	✔ ✔	✔ ✔ ✔	✔	✔ ✔ ✔
Stores straws or vials	✔	✔ ✔ ✔	✔ ✔	✔ ✔ ✔
Automatically filled	✔ ✔	✔ ✔ ✔	✔ ✔	N/A
Requires little monitoring or maintenance	✔ ✔ ✔	✔	✔	✔

Auditing

From time to time, the entire freezer inventory will require a systematic check through every sample stored, to reconcile these with the sperm bank records (and vice versa). Not only can this be a long and laborious task, but it is also a hazardous one for both operators and samples (Tomlinson & Morroll, 2008). In liquid-phase storage, the narrow vessel neck means that samples cannot be checked unless they are completely removed. The risk of premature thawing can be reduced by transferring the samples to a smaller flask on the bench-top to keep them bathed in nitrogen while their identifying information is verified. Auditing can be much simpler and safer in a large nitrogen vapor refrigerator with a wide lid area. Although this does contribute to the heavy nitrogen consumption of these vessels, it does permit checking of either straws or vials *in situ*. Placing an aluminium tray across the inventory (Figure 7.9) can make this task even simpler by helping to maintain very low temperatures as well as reducing the risk of losing a straw or vial at the bottom of the freezer.

Staff safety

The risks to both staff working within the sperm bank and the specimens in their custody are considerable, and should not be underestimated. Injury to personnel, sample loss, premature sample thaw, and the transmission of infectious disease between samples, though thankfully rare, are all potentially very costly in terms of service user (clinician and patient) satisfaction or, indeed, litigation. The risks to staff were made very clear by an incident in Scotland resulting in the death of an experienced technician working in a sperm storage bank (www.news.bbc.co.uk/1/hi/scotland/484813.stm). Supply vessels should be regularly checked and serviced (gas supply companies are usually very helpful in this respect) and their movement throughout the building should be carefully controlled. Neither staff nor members of the public should accompany a vessel being transported to upper floors of a building in an elevator, for example. The building design must incorporate low-level

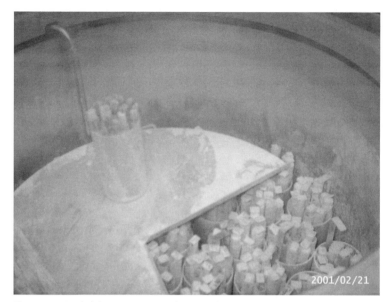
2001/02/21

Figure 7.9 Wide lid area on a vapor freezer with an aluminium tray, which is useful during audits and identification of samples by being able to hold individual goblets within the vapor at ultra-low temperatures.

extraction as well as oxygen-level monitoring, and this should be supported by regular equipment servicing, training in the use of all available personal protective equipment, and stringent procedures in case of failure. In the UK there are currently no requirements for any individual working in a sperm bank to receive even basic cryogenic training, either in the state or private sectors. UK professional bodies such as the Association of Biomedical Andrologists (ABA) (www.aba.uk.net) or the Association of Clinical Embryologists (ACE) (www.embryologists.org.uk) are discussing these issue with the government, other professional bodies, and the gas supply companies in order to standardize training to an accepted minimum level on a national basis.

Sample safety

In general, the risks to samples in long-term storage relate either to untimely thawing or transmission of viral and bacterial agents during storage. Untimely sample thawing is most likely to occur because the equipment or nitrogen supply has failed, or perhaps because sufficient care was not taken during straw or vial retrieval and identification. Supply failure could occur for many reasons, some of which have already been discussed, including the following.

- The pressurized vessel may fail or discharge its contents.
- Automated refrigerators may overfill and drain the vessel.
- The gas supply company may simply not deliver on time.

Such events could be overcome by providing contingency measures including:

- Extra capacity in terms of nitrogen delivery vessels.
- Appropriate written procedures.
- Training for all relevant staff.

Loss of coolant caused by vessel vacuum failure is, thankfully, a rare event that nevertheless requires consideration as part of a risk management strategy. Vacuum failure may be slow over a number of years, as in an aged and failing vessel, or it may be an acute event that is largely unpredictable and is just as likely to occur in a new vessel as it is in an old one. Provided that an appropriate monitoring and alarm system is in place (see below) to detect any untoward events, suitably qualified sperm bank staff should have a chance to respond and save samples from thawing. Clearly, this may not always be possible and additional risk reduction measures should be in place to minimize losses, including the provision of spare vessels and reducing risk by storing each patient's samples in two (or more) vessels.

Early warning and monitoring

Sperm banks owe a "duty of care" to their clients and must install some form of early-warning system in order to detect any malfunctions such as increases in temperature, reduction in the level of liquid nitrogen in storage vessels, or depletion of oxygen in the sperm bank. Each of these problems may be detected with the aid of an appropriate sensor linked to some form of alarm. Monitoring the liquid level is more suitable for dewars than temperature sensors since they will remain extremely cold with only a very small amount of liquid within them and the alarm may sound too late for any action to be taken. Alarms may be linked to a local bleeper, beacon, an automated telephone call, or a warning system linked to other devices within the organization such as a fire panel or a permanently staffed control room to alert staff out of hours. Obviously, there is little point in having a sophisticated system and not providing the appropriate cover necessary to answer any call. To reduce callouts, many sperm banks have now installed comprehensive monitoring systems, which not only provide early warning in emergency situations but also provide continuous data-logging of vital equipment and a remote call-in facility for interrogating and diagnosing any fault.

Theoretically, monitoring may then take place from almost anywhere providing the software is installed on a portable personal computer and an appropriate mobile telephone link-up is available. Remote interrogation of a system not only provides reassurance for the laboratory but also means that, with appropriate management, false alarms are dealt with in an instant and emergency site visits are kept to a minimum.

Summary and conclusions

It is quite likely that in the future, chemotherapeutic regimens with reduced toxicity and better-targeted radiotherapy will significantly reduce the demand for sperm banking. For the time being, however, it remains the only realistic option for the preservation of fertility in men receiving cytotoxic treatments. As ICSI has revolutionized the treatment of male factor infertility (see Chapter 8), and most men who freeze and store sperm now have a realistic chance of initiating a pregnancy providing their sperm are still viable, it is clear that many sperm banks feel that they have fulfilled their obligation to patients simply by providing a service. However, there is always room for improvement and sperm banks should regularly review their procedures for processing, freezing, and storing samples long-term for later use in assisted reproduction procedures. At the same time, careful consideration of storage-associated risks is required, in particularly those relating to the well-being of staff and samples.

References

Ackerman, D.R. (1968). Damage to human spermatozoa during storage at warming temperatures. *International Journal of Fertility*, **13**, 220–5.

Alvarez, J.G. & Storey B.T. (1993). Evidence that membrane stress contributes more than lipid peroxidation to sublethal cryodamage in cryopreserved human sperm: glycerol and other polyols as sole cryoprotectant. *Journal of Andrology*, **14**, 199–209.

Barkey, J., Zuckerman, H. & Heiman, M.A. (1974). A new, practical method of freezing and storing human sperm and a preliminary report on its use. *Fertility and Sterility*, **25**, 399–406.

Behrman, S.J. & Ackerman, D.R. (1969). Freeze preservation of human sperm. *American Journal of Obstetrics and Gynecology*, **103**, 654–64.

Clarke, G. (1999). Sperm cryopreservation: is there a significant risk of cross-contamination? *Human Reproduction*, **14**, 2941–3.

Donnelly, E.T., Steele, E.K., McClure, N. & Lewis, S.E. (2001). Assessment of DNA integrity and morphology of ejaculated spermatozoa from fertile and infertile men before and after cryopreservation. *Human Reproduction*, **16**, 1191–9.

Esteves, S.C., Sharma, R.K., Thomas, A.J. & Agarwal, A. (2000). Improvement in motion characteristics and acrosome status in cryopreserved human spermatozoa by swim-up processing before freezing. *Human Reproduction*, **15**, 2173–9.

Fountain, D., Ralston, M., Higgins, N. *et al.* (1997). Liquid nitrogen freezers: a potential source of microbial contamination of hematopoietic stem cell components. *Transfusion*, **37**, 585–91.

Gao, D.Y., Liu, J., Liu, C. *et al.* (1995). Prevention of osmotic injury to human spermatozoa during addition and removal of glycerol. *Human Reproduction*, **10**, 1109–22.

Human Fertilisation and Embryology Authority (HFEA). (2007). Procurement, processing, storage and handling of gametes and embryos. In *Code of Practice*, 7th ed. London: HFEA, p. G9.4.

Kim, L.U., Johnson, M.R., Barton, S. *et al.* (1999). Evaluation of sperm washing as a potential method of reducing HIV transmission in HIV-discordant couples wishing to have children. *AIDS*, **16**, 645–51.

Matson, P. (1995). External quality assessment for semen analysis and sperm antibody detection: results of a pilot scheme. *Human Reproduction*, **10**, 620–5.

McLaughlin, E.A., Ford, W.C.L. & Hull, M.G. R. (1992). The contribution of the toxicity of glycerol–egg yolk citrate cryopreservative to the decline in human sperm motility during cryopreservation. *Journal of Reproduction and Fertility*, **95**, 749–54.

Meryman, H.T. (1963). Preservation of living cells. *Federation Proceedings*, **22**, 81–9.

Morris G.J., Acton, E. & Avery, S. (1999). A novel approach to sperm cryopreservation. *Human Reproduction*, **14**, 1013–21.

Morris, G.J., Acton, E., Faszer, K. *et al.* (2006). Cryopreservation of murine embryos, human spermatozoa and embryonic stem cells using a liquid nitrogen-free, controlled rate freezer. *Reproductive Biomedicine Online*, **13**, 421–6.

Mortimer, D. (2004). Symposium: Cryopreservation and assisted human conception – current and future concepts and practices in human sperm cryobanking. *Reproductive Biomedicine Online*, **9**, 134–51.

NHS Executive (1997). *Guidance Notes on the Processing, Storage and Issue of Bone Marrow and Blood Stem Cells*. London: Department of Health.

Nicopoullos, J.D., Frodsham, L.C., Ramsay, J. W. *et al.* (2004). Synchronous sperm retrieval and sperm washing in an intracytoplasmic sperm injection cycle in an azoospermic man who was positive for human immunodeficiency virus. *Fertility and Sterility*, **81**, 670–4.

Nunc. (2003). *Safety First. Nunc Cryopreservation Manual*. Rochester, NY: Nalge Nunc International.

Paras, L., Freisinger, J., Esterbauer, B. *et al.* (2007). Cryopreservation technique: comparison of test yolk buffer versus SpermCryo and vapour versus computerised freezing. *Andrologia*, **40**, 18–22.

Ragni, G., Caccamo, A.M., Dalla Serra, A. & Guercilena, S. (1990). Computerized slow-stage freezing of semen from men with testicular tumours or Hodgkin's disease preserves sperm better than standard vapor freezing. *Fertility and Sterility*, **53**, 1072–5.

Saritha, K.R. & Bongso, A. (2001). Comparative evaluation of fresh and washed human sperm cryopreserved in vapour and liquid phases of liquid nitrogen. *Journal of Andrology*, **22**, 857–62.

Sharma, R.K. & Agarwal, A. (1997). Influence of artificial stimulation on unprocessed and Percoll-washed cryopreserved sperm. *Archives of Andrology*, **38**, 173–9.

Sherman, J.K. (1973). Synopsis of the use of frozen human sperm since 1964: state of art of human sperm banking. *Fertility and Sterility*, **24**, 397–412.

Smith, K.D. & Steinberger, E. (1973). Survival of spermatozoa in a human sperm bank. Effects of long-term storage in liquid nitrogen. *Journal of the American Medical Association*, **223**, 774–7.

Tedder, R.S., Zuckerman, M.A., Goldstone, A.H. *et al.* (1995). Hepatitis B transmission from contaminated cryopreservation tank. *Lancet*, **15**, 137–40.

Tomlinson, M.J. (2005). Opinion: Managing risk associated with cryopreservation. *Human Reproduction*, **20**, 1751–6.

Tomlinson, M.J. & Barratt, C.L.R. (2004). Donor insemination. In P. Sernal & C. Overton, eds., *Good Clinical Practice in Assisted Conception*. Cambridge: Cambridge University Press, pp. 86–99.

Tomlinson, M.J. & Morroll, D. (2008) Risks associated with cryopreservation: a survey of assisted conception units in the UK and Ireland. *Human Fertility*, **11**, 33–42.

World Health Organization (1999). *WHO Laboratory Manual for the Examination of Human Semen and Sperm–Cervical Mucus Interaction*, 4th edn. Cambridge: Cambridge University Press.

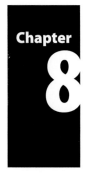

Chapter 8

Assisted reproduction using banked sperm

Hasan M. El-Fakahany and Denny Sakkas

Introduction

Although sperm banking is widely offered prior to the administration of potentially gonadotoxic therapies (see Chapter 2), few studies have systematically examined the natural fertility of men in the years following the end of treatment. While it has been shown that relatively few men with banked sperm actually use their samples in assisted conception treatment (see below), it is not known whether this is because their natural fertility has recovered sufficiently for them to conceive naturally or for other reasons. This chapter will examine the data on posttreatment fertility and guide the reader through the various options for assisted conception with banked sperm should natural fertility not recover.

Natural fertility after gonadotoxic therapy

The recovery (or maintenance) of natural fertility after gonadotoxic therapy is perhaps best observed through an assessment of semen quality posttreatment. Bahadur *et al.* (2005) found that, after treatment for a variety of cancers, only 37 percent of patients had permanent posttreatment azoospermia after a mean follow-up period of 48.6 months (see Table 8.1). Interestingly, the type of cancer (or disease) and the initial pretreatment sperm concentration were the most significant factors governing posttreatment semen quality and the recovery of spermatogenesis. For example, patients with lymphoma and leukemia had the highest incidence of posttreatment azoospermia and oligozoospermia, but while men with testicular cancer had the lowest pre-treatment sperm concentrations they also had the lowest incidence of azoospermia after treatment. This confirms the observation of Lampe *et al.* (1997), who found that in 170 men diagnosed with testicular cancer (treated with orchidectomy and cisplatin-based chemotherapy) only 20 percent were azoospermic one year after the end of treatment and there was evidence of continued improvement for up to five years.

With regard to pregnancy data, Herr *et al.* (1998) showed that, over a 10-year follow-up period of men with stage I testis tumor, 65 percent of couples who attempted a pregnancy were successful. More recently, a study by Brydøy *et al.* (2005) of 1814 men previously diagnosed with testicular cancer found that the 15-year actuarial posttreatment paternity rate was 71 percent without the use of cryopreserved sperm. Similarly, Magelssen *et al.* (2005) showed that 63 percent of male cancer patients ($n = 463$) had become a father by the age of 35 compared with 64 percent of men in the general population ($n = 367068$) who had not been treated with gonadotoxic agents. Despite such positive outcomes, it remains the case that for some treatments (e.g. total body irradiation) the rate of spontaneous pregnancy is known to be very low, with isolated pregnancies reported (Pakkala *et al.*, 1994; Check *et al.*, 2000).

Sperm Banking: Theory and Practice, eds. Allan A. Pacey and Mathew J. Tomlinson.
Published by Cambridge University Press. © Cambridge University Press 2009.

Table 8.1 *Incidence of posttreatment azoospermia (no sperm in the ejaculate), oligozoospermia (< 20 million sperm per mL) and normozoospermia (> 20 million sperm per mL) in 314 men treated with gonadotoxic therapy*

		Sperm concentration ($\times 10^6$ per mL) (%)		
Diagnosis	*n*	0	<20	>20
Leukemia	13	46	8	46
Lymphoma	128	58	14	27
Testicular cancer	102	12	38	50
Benign condition	13	16	23	61
Other malignant neoplasms	58	34	33	33

Table 8.2 *Summary of reports outlining the use of banked sperm in assisted conception procedures*

Diagnosis	No. of men banked	Follow-up (years)	Usage (%)	Reference
Mixed	833	22	7.0–9.0	Kelleher *et al.* (2001)
Hodgkin's disease	122	10.1	27.0	Blackhall *et al.* (2002)
Mixed	318	N/A	9.1	Agarwal *et al.* (2004)
Testicular	422	5.16	7.0	Magelssen *et al.* (2005)

Use of banked sperm in assisted conception

The first birth after freezing human spermatozoa with glycerol in liquid nitrogen vapor was reported by Perloff *et al.* (1964). The subsequent development of human sperm cryobanks in the 1970s gave rise to a growing use of sperm banking for patients receiving cytotoxic therapy. The first pregnancies and births following the use of sperm banked prior to cancer treatment reported a total of 117 pregnancies and 115 births (Sanger *et al.*, 1992). However, in spite of these early successes, current evidence indicates that, of the many men who store sperm, only a small proportion (10–25 percent) ever request to attempt pregnancy with their frozen samples (see Table 8.2). This may be a reflection of the relatively good fertility rates observed after potentially gonadotoxic therapy (see above) or, equally, may reflect poor access to (or funding of) assisted conception services. What is clear is that such analyses are based on historical datasets and that, as recently as the early 1990s, men may be denied access to sperm banking unless they had normal or near-normal semen parameters, as the subsequent treatment options for their thawed sperm were severely limited. However, the development of intracytoplasmic sperm injection (ICSI) initiated a considerable interest in banking sperm from men who have poor initial semen quality (Polcz *et al.*, 1998). Although cryopreservation and subsequent thawing are associated with a variable loss of sperm viability and motility, poor semen quality has not been shown to affect fertilization or pregnancy rates after cryopreservation and in vitro fertilization (IVF) or ICSI, as long as live sperm can be recovered (Kuczyński *et al.*, 2001).

Techniques of assisted conception

Several assisted conception techniques are available for use with banked sperm, or in cases where low levels of sperm production is occurring posttreatment, and assisted conception is still required with freshly ejaculated or surgically retrieved sperm (see Chapter 6). These are outlined in more detail below.

Intrauterine insemination

Early techniques of assisted conception involved inseminating fresh or frozen or thawed sperm into the vagina of the man's partner using a syringe or catheter. Although such intracervical insemination is very easy to perform, and associated with low morbidity, the success rates are largely dependent on the quality of the sample being inseminated and therefore limited to only the better-quality samples (fresh or frozen). Following the development of new sperm preparation methods in the 1980s, during which sperm could reliably be separated from the components of seminal plasma (Mortimer, 1994), alternative insemination strategies could be attempted. As a consequence, concentrated preparations of sperm were inseminated directly into the Fallopian tubes, peritoneal cavity, or ovarian follicles of women, before a consensus that transvaginal intrauterine insemination (IUI) was the most effective method was finally reached, providing an optimum chance of conception combined with the lowest rate of complications (Sacks & Simon, 1991). Although IUI may be performed on women in the natural cycle, it is now almost always combined with some element of ovarian stimulation to increase the success rates (Guzick et al., 1999).

In vitro fertilization

Following the birth of the world's first IVF baby in 1978 (Steptoe & Edwards, 1978), it has been estimated that worldwide more than three million babies have been born using the procedure (ESHRE, 2006). The process of IVF is relatively straightforward and indeed technically relatively routine (see Braude & Rowell, 2006).

Briefly, in an IVF cycle the female partner is given stimulatory drugs (usually gonado-trophins) in the weeks leading up to the procedure, to trigger the development of a number of ovarian follicles that can be collected for fertilization in the laboratory. Egg collection is performed under sedation, with each ovarian follicle being punctured by a needle and the contents aspirated into a tube. These follicular fluids are examined in the laboratory, and any eggs recovered are incubated with sperm obtained either from a fresh masturbatory sample or from a sample that has been previously frozen (see above) or surgically recovered (see Chapter 6). Sperm are prepared for co-incubation with oocytes in the same manner described for IUI (above) and are incubated with eggs for up to 24 hours in culture dishes maintained in an incubator at 37°C and 5 percent CO_2. Typically, 60–70 percent of eggs recovered are fertilized and the majority will develop into embryos (Figure 8.1). Embryo transfer into the uterine cavity usually occurs on the second or third day after egg collection, with any excess embryos being frozen for transfer at a later date if required. Success rates (clinical pregnancies) with IVF across Europe are typically 26.1 percent per egg collection and 29.6 percent per embryo transfer, respectively, (Andersen et al., 2007), although success rates decline markedly for females over the age of 35 (HFEA, 2005).

For IVF to work effectively, up to a hundred thousand sperm need to be incubated with each oocyte in order to be sure that fertilization will occur (Elder & Dale, 2000). Therefore,

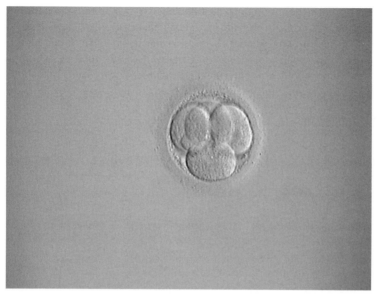

Figure 8.1 A human embryo at the four-cell stage following fertilization of a human oocyte in vitro.

for ejaculates or banked sperm from which several million sperm cannot be recovered or collected, traditional IVF is not an effective option and ICSI needs to be attempted.

Intracytoplasmic sperm injection

In an attempt to improve in vitro fertilization rates for men with low sperm counts, or in situations where sperm had poor or no motility, many research groups in the late 1980s tried a number of strategies to facilitate the entry of weakly or immotile sperm through the zona pellucida of eggs during IVF. These include zona drilling (ZD), partial zona dissection (PZD), and subzonal insemination (SUZI). ICSI arose from an accident during a SUZI procedure, where the pipette containing the sperm pierced the oolemma (rather than leaving it in the perivitelline space) and introduced the sperm directly into the egg cytoplasm (Figure 8.2). Surprisingly, the egg fertilized and an embryo developed. Moreover, when the embryo was transferred to the woman a normal pregnancy resulted (Palermo *et al.*, 1992). ICSI now accounts for over 50 percent of all in vitro fertilization procedures in many clinics and has universally revolutionized the treatment of male infertility as a consequence. The clinical pregnancy rates by use of ICSI are very similar to those observed with IVF, at 26.5 percent per egg collection and 28.7 percent per embryo transfer, respectively (Andersen *et al.*, 2007).

Choice of assisted conception technique

The choice of assisted conception technique for the patient with banked sperm will depend on a number of factors, including:

- Quality (and quantity) of the sperm available (freshly ejaculated or cryopreserved).
- Physiology and assumed fertility of the female partner.
- Choice of patient.
- Funding available to the patient.

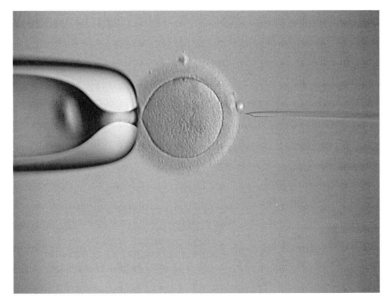

Figure 8.2 A human oocyte, with the cumulus cells removed and held in place by a holding pipette (left) immediately prior to injection with a fine needle (right) containing a human sperm (not visible).

This is summarized in Figure 8.3. In most cases, the sperm bank will have advised at the outset the kind of assisted conception options which might be available to the couple, that is, whether the banked samples might be sufficient in number and/or quality to attempt IUI in a female partner with normal reproductive physiology; or, whether ICSI will remain the only option available because the banked samples are too poor to contemplate anything else. At the time of sperm banking this is a difficult discussion for the patient, but it is useful information that should be provided.

Several studies have been performed on evaluating the use of cryopreserved sperm in assisted conception, especially in patients banking sperm before treatment for a malignancy. For example, Rosenlund *et al.* (1998) reported the outcome from 15 couples undergoing assisted conception with banked sperm because of previous testicular cancer in the male partner. The couples underwent a total of 7 IVF cycles and 11 ICSI cycles resulting in 12 pregnancies. In 1998, Lass *et al.* (1998) described the outcome in 6 couples undergoing assisted conception following chemotherapy in the male using banked sperm: 2 couples achieved a pregnancy after IUI, 1 couple after IVF, and 2 after ICSI. Another study reported that, out of 258 men who had their semen banked owing to cancer treatment, only 18 returned for treatment, resulting in 6 pregnancies (Audrins *et al.*, 1999). Ginsburg *et al.* (2001) evaluated the results in an IVF program enrolling cancer patients of which 19 were men whom, together with their partners, underwent a total of 35 cycles. A total of 11 of these cycles used banked sperm, resulting in 3 pregnancies, while the remaining 24 cycles used fresh sperm, resulting in 11 pregnancies, thereby giving a pregnancy rate of 40 percent per cycle. Recently, Agarwal *et al.* (2004) reported the outcome of assisted reproductive techniques (ART) in 29 male cancer survivors, all using cryopreserved semen. Almost 40 percent of the patients were able to achieve a healthy live birth. A total of 87 cycles were performed with a mean pregnancy rate of 18.3 percent per cycle (7 percent after IUI, 23 percent after IVF, and 37 percent after ICSI). Schmidt *et al.* (2004) followed the fertility outcome in a consecutive series of 67 couples referred for ART from 1996 to 2003

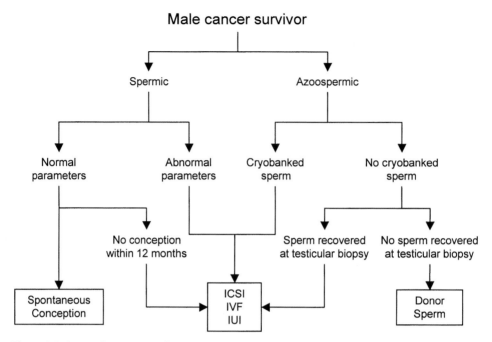

Figure 8.3 Options for conception for male patients who have undergone sperm banking prior to potentially sterilizing treatments. The options available may be natural conception or assisted conception depending on the quality of sperm available (fresh or frozen).

because of a previous cancer diagnosis in the male. They reported a pregnancy rate of 14.8 percent after IUI and 38.6 percent after ICSI using banked sperm.

Using fresh or frozen sperm in assisted conception?

A common question posed prior to assisted conception when there is an option of using either banked sperm or freshly ejaculated (or surgically recovered) sperm posttreatment (i.e. when some spermatogenesis is still occurring after gonadotoxic therapy) is: Which sperm to use? This is asked because of concern for the possibility of significant sperm DNA damage occurring in either type of sample. Ironically, sperm DNA damage may arise from the cryopreservation process used to bank sperm or as a consequence of gonadotoxic therapy.

In the case of the cryopreservation process, Donnelly *et al.* (2001) identified a significant decrease – of 20 percent – in the DNA integrity of sperm after cryopreservation in the sperm from men with poor semen quality. Interestingly, the sperm DNA from fertile men with normal semen quality was unaffected by sperm cryopreservation. Therefore, since the semen quality of men with cancer may be impaired prior to treatment (see Chapter 6), this may lead to higher levels of sperm DNA damage than is evident in men from the general population.

With regard to treatment-related DNA damage, Ståhl *et al.* (2006) examined 96 men with testicular cancer, from whom semen was collected at specific intervals until five years after treatment. Sperm DNA integrity in men postsurgery (orchidectomy) did not differ significantly from the control group. However, compared with pretreatment values, radiotherapy induced a transient increase in sperm DNA damage, but this returned to normal levels after three to five years. Ståhl *et al.* (2006) concluded that irradiation increased sperm DNA damage for one to two years after treatment, and 38 percent of irradiated patients with normozoospermia had high (> 27 percent) DNA damage, which could affect sperm-fertilizing ability.

Damage to sperm DNA strongly correlates with mutagenic events (Twigg *et al.*, 1998). However, sperm with damaged genetic material are still capable of fertilization and defects may not become evident until the embryo has divided or the fetus has developed (reviewed by Seli & Sakkas, 2005). Poor-quality sperm are known to contain partially decondensed chromatin that is associated with DNA strand breaks and may make them more susceptible to freezing. Sperm DNA damage after spermiogenesis will be irrevocable, regardless of whether it transpires during storage in the epididymis, after ejaculation in the female reproductive tract, or during processing for use in assisted reproduction. Hence, any damage imposed on sperm DNA by the freezing and thawing process will remain throughout the insemination procedure and beyond. Therefore, freezing sperm in a way that provides maximum protection to DNA is vital to prevent the possible conveyance of damage to offspring (Donnelly *et al.*, 2001).

Tests of DNA quality and sperm selection methods

To assist reproductive biologists, a number of tests have been developed in recent years to measure sperm DNA quality. These include the terminal deoxynucleotidyl transferase (TdT)-mediated dUTP nick end-labeling (TUNEL) assay (Sun *et al.*, 1997), in situ nick translation (Tomlinson *et al.*, 2001), single-cell electrophoresis and the comet assay (Morris *et al.*, 2002), or the sperm chromatin structure assay (Evenson *et al.*, 1999). However, although there are many papers outlining their use in different clinical situations, there is currently no consensus concerning their clinical applicability (Practice Committee of the American Society for Reproductive Medicine, 2006).

Using the above tests, it has been shown that washing sperm samples by the density gradient centrifugation technique can significantly enrich the number of sperm with undamaged DNA in the washed preparation (Tomlinson *et al.*, 2001). Sakkas *et al.* (2000) showed that there was a significant ($p < 0.001$) decrease in both chromomycin A3 (CMA3) positivity (which indirectly demonstrates the presence of protamines) and DNA strand breakage in sperm samples from different men after preparation by density gradient centrifugation. Similarly, Ainsworth *et al.* (2005) have developed a novel electrophoretic sperm isolation technique for the isolation of functional human spermatozoa free from significant DNA damage. Briefly, the separation system consists of a cassette comprising two chambers: semen is introduced into one chamber and a current applied leading to a purified suspension of spermatozoa collecting in the other. Sperm suspensions generated by the electrophoretic separation technique contain motile, viable, morphologically normal spermatozoa that exhibit lower levels of DNA damage. Subsequently, Ainsworth *et al.* (2007) reported the first pregnancy, and normal birth, using sperm isolated using this technique.

A different approach has been developed by Huszar and collaborators (Huszar *et al.*, 2003), who exploited the observation that sperm that are able to bind to hyaluronic acid (HA) are mature and have completed the spermiogenetic process of sperm plasma membrane remodeling, cytoplasmic extrusion, and nuclear histone–protamine replacement. DNA testing of the sperm selected by this method showed that the chromosomal disomy frequencies were reduced from 0.52 to 0.16 percent, diploidy from 0.51 to 0.09 percent, and sex chromosome disomy from 0.27 to 0.05 percent in comparison with the control (unbound) sperm. They concluded that the ICSI sperm selection method could reduce the potential genetic complications and adverse public health effects of ICSI (Jakab *et al.*, 2005).

Finally, Bartoov *et al.* (2001) used high-magnification microscopy to select the sperm for injection in the ICSI procedure based on the morphology of the sperm nucleus. They reported that by use of this method they were able to achieve a pregnancy rate of 58 percent in patients who had previously failed at least five consecutive routine cycles of IVF and ICSI. They also reported, in a follow-up study (Bartoov *et al.*, 2003), an improvement in pregnancy rates with ICSI and morphologically selected sperm compared with conventional ICSI.

Ultimately, selection of the most appropriate ART and whether it uses the patient's fresh or frozen samples will be a careful balancing act for the team providing assisted conception. They must assess the relative risk of genetic anomaly resulting from cryopreservation against enduring DNA anomalies if spermatogenesis has resumed, and estimate which is most likely to give the desired outcome: a healthy baby.

Case reports

It is now been shown that banked sperm can survive and retain their ability to fertilize after many years of storage. For example, Horne *et al.* (2004) reported a live birth following ICSI treatment using sperm that had been banked for a total of 21 years. Similarly, Feldschuh *et al.* (2005) reported two pregnancies after successful IUI following sperm banking for 28 years. Clearly, such events will become more commonplace in years to come, and illustrate the effectiveness of sperm banking procedures in preserving male fertility.

Conclusions

Sperm banking has revolutionized the field of assisted reproduction following gonadotoxic therapy. There have been improvements both in the postthaw survival of banked sperm as well as the ART available to use low numbers of sperm from thawed samples or fresh ejaculates (e.g. ICSI). In general terms, it is always safer to use a banked (pregonadotoxic therapy) treatment sperm sample in assisted reproduction. Novel techniques that may allow a more stringent selection of spermatozoa will also help in facilitating the safety of treatment.

References

Agarwal, A., Ranganathan, P., Kattal, N. *et al.* (2004). Fertility after cancer: a prospective review of assisted reproductive outcome with banked semen specimens. *Fertility and Sterility*, **81**, 342–8.

Ainsworth, C., Nixon, B. & Aitken, R.J. (2005). Development of a novel electrophoretic system for the isolation of human spermatozoa. *Human Reproduction*, **20**, 2261–70.

Ainsworth, C., Nixon, B., Jansen, R.P. & Aitken, R.J. (2007). First recorded pregnancy and normal birth after ICSI using electrophoretically isolated spermatozoa. *Human Reproduction*, **22**, 197–200.

Andersen, A.N., Goossens, V., Gianaroli, L. *et al.* (2007). Assisted reproductive technology in Europe, 2003. Results generated from European registers by ESHRE. *Human Reproduction*, **22**, 1513–25.

Audrins, P., Holden, C.A., McLachlan, R.I. & Kovacs, G.T. (1999). Semen storage for special purposes at Monash IVF from 1977 to 1997. *Fertility and Sterility*, **72**, 179–81.

Bahadur, G., Nahadur, G., Ozturk, O. *et al.* (2005). Semen quality before and after gonadotoxic treatment. *Human Reproduction*, **20**, 774–81.

Bartoov, B., Berkovitz, A. & Eltes, F. (2001). Selection of spermatozoa with normal nuclei to improve the pregnancy rate with intracytoplasmic sperm injection.

New England Journal of Medicine, **345**, 1067–8.

Bartoov, B., Berkovitz, A., Eltes, F. *et al.* (2003). Pregnancy rates are higher with intracytoplasmic morphologically selected sperm injection than with conventional intracytoplasmic injection. *Fertility and Sterility*, **80**, 1413–19.

Blackhall, F.H., Atkinson, A.D., Maaya, M.B. *et al.* (2002), semen cryo preservation utilisation and reproductive outcome in men treated for Hodgkin's disease. *British Journal of Cancer*, **12**, 381–4.

Braude, P. & Rowell, P. (2006). Assisted conception II – In vitro fertilisation and intracytoplasmic sperm injection. *British Medical Journal*, **327**, 852–5.

Brydøy, M., Fosså, S.D., Klepp, O. *et al.* (2005). Paternity following treatment for testicular cancer. *Journal of the National Cancer Institute*, **97**, 1580–8.

Check, M.L., Brown, T. & Check, J.H. (2000). Recovery of spermatogenesis and successful conception after bone marrow transplant for acute leukaemia: case report. *Human Reproduction*, **15**, 83–5.

Donnelly, E.T., Steele, E.K., McClure, N. & Lewis, S.E. (2001). Assessment of DNA integrity and morphology of ejaculated spermatozoa from fertile and infertile men before and after cryopreservation. *Human Reproduction*, **16**, 1191–9.

Elder, K. & Dale, B. (2000). In Vitro *Fertilization*, 2nd edn. Cambridge: Cambridge University Press.

European Society of Human Reproduction and Embryology (ESHRE). (2006). "Three million babies born using assisted reproductive technologies." Press release at the 2006 Annual Meeting (available at www.eshre.com/emc.asp?pageId=806).

Evenson, D.P., Jost, L.K., Marshall, D. *et al.* (1999). Utility of the sperm chromatin structure assay as a diagnostic and prognostic tool in the human fertility clinic. *Human Reproduction*, **14**, 1039–49.

Feldschuh, J., Brassel, J., Durso, N. & Levine, A. (2005). Successful sperm storage for 28 years. *Fertility and Sterility*, **84**, 1017.

Ginsburg, E.S., Yanushpolsky, E.H. & Jackson, K.V. (2001). In vitro fertilization for cancer patients and survivors. *Fertility and Sterility*, **75**, 705–10.

Guzick, D.S., Carson, S.A., Coutifaris, C. *et al.* (1999). Efficacy of superovulation and intrauterine insemination in the treatment of infertility. National Cooperative Reproductive Medicine Network. *New England Journal of Medicine*, **340**, 177–83.

Herr, H.W., Bar-Chama, N., O'Sullivan, M. & Sogani, P.C. (1998). Paternity in men with stage I testis tumors on surveillance. *Journal of Clinical Oncology*, **16**, 733–4.

Horne, G., Atkinson, A.D., Pease, E.H. *et al.* (2004). Live birth with sperm cryopreserved for 21 years prior to cancer treatment: case report. *Human Reproduction*, **19**, 1448–9.

Human Fertilisation and Embryology Authority (HFEA). (2005). *The Patient's Guide*. London: HFEA.

Huszar, G., Ozenci, C.C., Cayli, S. *et al.* (2003). Hyaluronic acid binding by human sperm indicates cellular maturity, viability, and unreacted acrosomal status. *Fertility and Sterility*. **79**, 1616–24.

Jakab, A., Sakkas, D., Delpiano, E. *et al.* (2005). Intracytoplasmic sperm injection: a novel selection method for sperm with normal frequency of chromosomal aneuploidies. *Fertility and Sterility*, **84**, 1665–73.

Kelleher, S., Wishart, S.M., Liu, P.Y. *et al.* (2001). Long-term outcomes of elective human sperm cryostorage. *Human Reproduction*, **16**, 2632–9.

Kuczyński, W., Dhont, M., Grygoruk, C. *et al.* (2001). The outcome of intracytoplasmic injection of fresh and cryopreserved ejaculated spermatozoa – a prospective randomized study. *Human Reproduction*, **16**, 2109–13.

Lampe, H., Horwich, A., Norman, A., Nicholls, J. & Dearnaley, D.P. (1997). Fertility after chemotherapy for testicular germ cell cancers. *Journal of Clinical Oncology*, **15**, 239–45.

Lass, A., Akagbosu, F., Abusheikha, N. *et al.* (1998). A programme of semen cryopreservation for patients with malignant disease in a tertiary infertility centre: lessons from 8 years' experience. *Human Reproduction*, **13**, 3256–61.

Magelssen, H., Haugen, T.B., von Düring, V. *et al.* (2005). Twenty years, experience with semen cryopreservation in testicular cancer patients: who needs it? *European Urology*, **48**, 779–85.

Morris, I.D., Ilott, S., Dixon, L. & Brison, D.R. (2002). The spectrum of DNA damage in human sperm assessed by single cell gel electrophoresis (Comet assay) and its relationship to fertilization and embryo development. *Human Reproduction*, **17**, 990–8.

Mortimer, D. (1994). *Practical Laboratory Andrology*. New York, NY: Oxford University Press.

Pakkala, S., Lukka, M., Helminen, P., Koskimies, S. & Ruutu, T. (1994). Paternity after bone marrow transplantation following conditioning with total body irradiation. *Bone Marrow Transplantation*, **13**, 489–90.

Palermo, G., Joris, H., Devroey, P. & Van Steteghem, A.C. (1992). Pregnancies after intracytoplasmic sperm injection of a single spermatozoon into an oocyte. *Lancet*, **340**, 17–18.

Perloff, W.H., Steinberger, E. & Sherman, J.K. (1964). Conception with human spermatozoa frozen by nitrogen vapor technique. *Fertility and Sterility*, **15**, 501–4.

Polcz, T.E., Stronk, J., Xiong, C. et al. (1998). Optimal utilization of cryopreserved human semen for assisted reproduction: recovery and maintenance of sperm motility and viability. *Journal of Assisted Reproduction and Genetics*, **15**, 504–12.

Practice Committee of the American Society for Reproductive Medicine. (2006). The clinical utility of sperm DNA integrity testing. *Fertility and Sterility*, **86**, S35–7.

Rosenlund, B., Sjöblom, P., Törnblom, M., Hultling, C. & Hillensjö, T. (1998). In-vitro fertilization and intracytoplasmic sperm injection in the treatment of infertility after testicular cancer. *Human Reproduction*, **13**, 414–18.

Sacks, P.C. & Simon, J.A. (1991). Infectious complications of intrauterine insemination: a case report and literature review. *International Journal of Fertility*, **36**, 331–9.

Sakkas, D., Manicardi, G.C., Tomlinson, M. et al. (2000). The use of two density gradient centrifugation techniques and the swim-up method to separate spermatozoa with chromatin and nuclear DNA anomalies. *Human Reproduction*, **15**, 1112–16.

Sanger, W.G., Olson, J.H. & Sherman, J.K. (1992). Semen cryobanking for men with cancer – criteria change. *Fertility and Sterility*, **58**, 1024–7.

Schmidt, K.L., Larsen, E., Bangsbøll, S. et al. (2004). Assisted reproduction in male cancer survivors: fertility treatment and outcome in 67 couples. *Human Reproduction*, **19**, 2806–10.

Seli, E. & Sakkas, D. (2005). Spermatozoal nuclear determinants of reproductive outcome: implications for ART. *Human Reproduction Update*, **11**, 337–49.

Ståhl, O., Eberhard, J., Jepson, K. et al. (2006). Sperm DNA integrity in testicular cancer patients. *Human Reproduction*, **21**, 3199–205.

Steptoe, P.C. & Edwards, R.G. (1978). Birth after the re-implantation of a human embryo. *Lancet*, **2**, 366.

Sun, J.G., Jurisicova, A. & Casper, R.F. (1997). Detection of deoxyribonucleic acid fragmentation in human sperm: correlation with fertilization in vitro. *Biology of Reproduction*, **56**, 602–7.

Tomlinson, M.J., Moffatt, O., Manicardi, G.C. et al. (2001). Interrelationships between seminal parameters and sperm nuclear DNA damage before and after density gradient centrifugation: implications for assisted conception. *Human Reproduction*, **16**, 2160–5.

Twigg, J., Fulton, N., Gomez, E., Irvine, D.S. & Aitken, R.J. (1998). Analysis of the impact of intracellular reactive oxygen species generation on the structural and functional integrity of human spermatozoa: lipid peroxidation, DNA fragmentation and effectiveness of antioxidants. *Human Reproduction*, **13**, 1429–36.

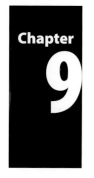

Chapter 9

Future developments for fertility preservation in men

Mathew J. Tomlinson and Allan A. Pacey

The previous chapters of this book have focussed on the practical aspects of providing sperm banking to men who face the threat of future infertility because of medical treatments. They illustrate how, in practical terms, sperm banking is now routine and can be highly effective at helping those who are able to provide a suitable sample for freezing prior to starting their treatment to become fathers. However, it is recognized that, for some, this may not be possible: either because they are too young (and have not gone through puberty), they are too ill at the time of their diagnosis to provide a semen sample, they do not have ready access to a suitable service, or the opportunity is not offered to them. For such individuals, it would be useful to have alternative approaches and this chapter concludes the book by summarizing the current research in this area. If successful, one or more of the following could revolutionize fertility preservation for males and provide an alternative to traditional sperm banking.

Pre- or posttreatment endocrine manipulation

Following the observation in women that gonadotrophin-releasing hormone (GnRH) analogs and antagonists might be able to spare the ovary from some of the harmful effects of chemotherapy and radiotherapy (see Mitwally, 2007 for review), similar approaches have been attempted in the male. If successful, such strategies could potentially lead to the restoration of natural fertility in a larger number of individuals without the need for sperm banking.

Although early experiments in the male were attempted with the aim of protecting against the loss of testicular stem cells during the cytotoxic insult, it soon became clear that the hormonal treatments probably enhanced the ability of the testis to maintain the differentiation of spermatozoa in the population of stem cells that survive treatment but which otherwise fail to differentiate once treatment has ended (Shetty & Meistrich, 2005). Since most of the experimental work to date has been performed on rats, it is unclear whether it can be adapted for human clinical application. Encouraging results from a small study of 15 patients with nephrotic syndrome (being treated with cyclophosphamide) have been obtained, although such treatments usually involve lower doses than those commonly used in the treatment of malignancies (Masala et al., 1997). More recent experiments in non-human primates (Boekelheide et al., 2005) have been unable to reproduce the experimental results obtained in rats, raising the possibility that there are important species-specific differences in the testicular response either to the treatment (in this case radiotherapy) or the endocrine rescue protocol, or both. More recently, Aminsharifi et al. (2007) suggested that the application of exogenous testosterone prior to cisplatin chemotherapy in the treatment of testicular cancer might be able to protect the gonad, but this remains to be

Sperm Banking: Theory and Practice, eds. Allan A. Pacey and Mathew J. Tomlinson. Published by Cambridge University Press. © Cambridge University Press 2009.

tested. Therefore, the use of endocrine manipulation to protect the testes from damage (or salvage them from it) is still very much experimental.

Freezing and retransplantation of gonadal tissue or cells posttreatment

Unlike the current approaches of freezing mature sperm, many authors have commented on the desirability of being able to remove (before treatment) and potentially replace (after treatment) sufficient gonadal tissue that might allow the patient subsequently to reproduce normally. Clearly, this would require the need for gonadal tissue to be frozen for a period of time (perhaps many years) and retain its viability when transplanted. The advantage of being able to do this is that, unlike frozen sperm that are a finite resource, stem cells in the testis are "self-renewing." Thus, if they could successfully be transplanted back into the patient, they could continue to produce sperm for the rest of his life. Even if this procedure was only moderately successful it could potentially provide sufficient (freshly ejaculated) sperm for use in repeated cycles of assisted conception. If very successful, and ejaculates were near normal in terms of quality, then it is possible to envisage some patients being able to father a child quite normally and without undergoing assisted conception.

Most progress has been made in the area of spermatogonial stem cell transplantation. Although this remained theoretical for many years, major progress was made when Brinster and Zimmermann (1994) published details of experiments where they had successfully removed spermatogonia from one mouse and transplanted them back into the testes of another. This provided proof that the technique was feasible, and the underlying technology for retrieval, storage, and transplantation of spermatogonia has been developed in subsequent years (see Johnson et al., 2000). Using a mouse experimental model, Nagano et al. (2002) found that stem cell colonization into the testis was not influenced by cryopreservation of donor cells or donor cell concentration, suggesting that stem cells could survive long-term storage. Moreover, Kantasu-Shinohara et al. (2003) further demonstrated that the restoration of fertility in infertile male mice could be achieved by the transplantation of cryopreserved spermatogonia from fertile mouse donors. Somewhat understandably, scientists have been notably cautious with progress to human clinical trials and, although some small-scale trials have been attempted (Radford et al., 1999), at the time of writing, the results have not yet been published.

An obvious concern with retransplantation of gonadal tissue is in the fear that during the process malignant cells may be reintroduced into the patient who was otherwise cured of his original disease. It has been suggested that this is particularly pertinent for lymphoma and leukemia patients, as in these diseases the testis is a likely organ for the settlement of metastasizing cells (Schlatt, 2002), as has been shown experimentally in leukemic rats (Jahnukainen et al., 2001). Ellen and Herman (2007) have recently discussed this issue and suggested a number of possible decontamination strategies that could be employed. However, at present there is too little information about such risks to adequately advise patients and it is clear that only following large-scale studies could this be properly evaluated.

Sperm production in vitro

As an alternative to spermatogonial stem cell transplantation, the development of in vitro culture technology might, in theory, allow spermatogenesis to be supported in the laboratory to a sufficient level that mature sperm might be produced to be used in in vitro fertilization (IVF) or intracytoplasmic sperm injection (ICSI) procedures. This would obviously remove the concern of reintroducing cancerous cells back into the patient, as outlined above.

The prospects for spermatogenesis in vitro have recently been reviewed by Parks *et al.* (2003), who outlined the technical complexity of cell-culture systems that would be required to maintain the development of spermatozoa in vitro. More recently, Huleihel *et al.* (2007) reviewed the current obstacles and pointed to the recent identification of testicular paracrine or autocrine factors, and specific molecular markers of spermatogonial stem cells, that have allowed some progress to be made. Even so, while some groups have succeeded in the in vitro culture of spermtogonial stem cells, only presumptive spermatids expressing appropriate genetic markers have been identified and have been injected into eggs to produce viable embryos. It is far from the stage of being clinically useful for human applications. There is obvious concern about whether or not sperm produced in vitro will still undergo all the genetic and epigenetic alterations that the male gamete normally undergoes during in vivo spermatogenesis (Georgiou *et al.*, 2007). If this is not the case, then any use of such sperm in assisted reproductive technology may lead to poor outcome, but also more worryingly potential health consequences for any children born.

Xenotransplantation of reproductive tissues

Many research groups have been developing techniques to transplant gonadal tissue into a "host" animal that could act to support the development of sperm to the point that they might be harvested and used in IVF or ICSI. Proof of principle has been demonstrated through experiments dating back to the 1970s that illustrate the potential for testicular tissue or isolated spermatogonial stem cells to be transplanted from one species to another and for spermatogenesis to be supported in the host animal (reviewed by Parks *et al.*, 2003). For example, Honaramooz *et al.* (2002) demonstrated that pieces of testicular tissue from immature rhesus monkeys (*Macaca mulatta*) could be grafted to an ectopic site (under the skin) of immunodeficient castrated nude mice, as xenografts. The grafted tissue was revascularized in the ectopic site and showed complete spermatogenesis, producing fertilization-competent sperm. In a later experiment, Schlatt *et al.* (2003) demonstrated the birth of live progeny from the ectopic grafting of neonatal mouse testes using a similar approach.

Although such approaches have been pivotal in furthering our understanding of the biology of spermatogenesis (Dobrinski, 2005), they also open up the avenue for fertility preservation strategies. Primarily, this might be seen as a method of generating sperm from tissue taken from postpubertal individuals before cancer treatment, but it has also been suggested that this may give hope for fertility preservation in prepubertal boys where traditional sperm banking is not possible. A recent study by Wyns *et al.* (2007) demonstrated that tissue taken from the cryptorchid testis of young boys (aged between 2 and 12 years old) could be successfully frozen and subsequently grafted into the scrotum of mice to support the survival and proliferative activity of spermatogonia and Sertoli cells.

While the xenotransplantation of gonadal tissue currently has many research applications, its use as a method of generating gametes for human reproductive application raises many ethical concerns (Cozzi *et al.*, 2006). There are obvious safety concerns to address about the potential for nonhuman DNA (or animal viruses) being transferred to the human genome during the assisted conception procedure, and thus much work is also needed to establish the safety and acceptability of this approach.

Generation of artificial sperm

In the absence of any frozen testicular tissue or sperm, it has been proposed that two options for the generation of artificial sperm might be possible to overcome infertility in those men where sperm banking was not possible. The first is based upon an approach for in vitro haploidization of somatic cells to produce sperm-like cells that could be used in ICSI procedures. In 2003, Tesarik and Mendoza discussed an approach whereby a somatic cell nucleus could be injected into an oocyte (without previous enucleation), and somatic nucleus haploidization would occur in the presence of the original female nucleus (triploid-to-diploid reduction), it was hoped leading to the formation of a diploid embryo (Tesarik & Mendoza, 2003). An alternative approach taken by Toyooka *et al.* (2003) and Geijsen *et al.* (2004) showed that sperm-like cells could be generated from mouse embryonic stem cells cultured in the laboratory. Similarly, Drusenheimer *et al.* (2007) suggested that cells in human bone marrow may potentially differentiate into male germ cell-like cells, as shown by the expression of early germ cell markers and male germ cell specific markers. Clearly, there are ethical and safety concerns to consider before using such an approach and, in a more recent report, Nayernia *et al.* (2006) showed that although sperm-like cells (created from embryonic stem cells) could induce normal development and live pups when injected into mouse eggs, the pups were unhealthy and died prematurely. The concern about the safety aspects of generating artificial gametes for human applications was recently highlighted by the UK Government, which proposes to make their use in assisted conception illegal in a forthcoming revision of the fertility laws in the UK (DoH, 2006).

Alternatives to cold storage in liquid nitrogen

Although the above discussions concentrate on alternative approaches for fertility preservation that do not rely upon the storage of ejaculated sperm, some technical progress has been made in the storage of sperm without the need for cold temperatures. Wakyama and Yanagimachi (1998) reported the remarkable discovery showing that freeze-dried mouse sperm had the full developmental potential to generate healthy offspring when injected into mouse eggs. This discovery led to similar reports in rabbits (Liu *et al.*, 2004) and rats (Hochi *et al.*, 2008). Although little work to date has been done on human sperm, Kusakabe *et al.* (2007) have shown that the chromosomes of both mouse and human sperm are undamaged by freeze-drying, thereby opening the possibility that this technique might be applicable to fertility preservation in the human male. If it were successful then this could radically change the nature of sperm banks. It would remove the need for storing sperm in liquid nitrogen, with the dangers that this poses to staff (see Chapter 7), and it would make transferring sperm from one sperm bank to another much easier and cheaper.

Reduction in toxicity of chemotherapy regimens

Advances in chemotherapy since the mid 1990s has focussed not only on improved patient survival but also on reducing toxic side effects, including those affecting reproductive function. Clearly, by reducing the toxicity of therapies used for either malignant or non-malignant diseases, the requirement for sperm banking could also be reduced. In many cases drug regimens remain highly toxic, in particular those using large doses of alkylating agents, and sperm banking would be recommended without question. Yet, for certain diagnoses, alternative drugs and regimens have been introduced successfully and fertility has remained intact for many. The most obvious example is perhaps that of the treatment for Hodgkin's lymphoma. Previously, these patients may have received either chlorambucil, vinblastine, procarbazine, prednisolone, doxorubicin, vincristine, etoposide, bleomycin (ChIVPP/PABIOE) or mechlorethamine, vincristine, procarbazine, prednisolone, adriamycin, bleomycin, vinblastine (MOPP/ABV), both of which exhibit significant toxicity (Chapman *et al.*, 1979; Canellos *et al.*, 1992; Bokemeyer, *et al.*, 1996; Ben Arush *et al.*, 2000). In more recent years patients with Hodgkin's lymphoma (stages IB, IIB, III, and IV) have preferably been treated with the combination chemotherapy regimen adriamycin, bleomycin, vincristine, dacarbazine (ABVD) with apparently reduced toxicity (Bonadonna, 1982; Viviani *et al.*, 1985; Anselmo *et al.*, 1990; Tal *et al.*, 2000). Interest was first generated by Viviani and colleagues (1985), who compared six cycles of MOPP ($n = 29$) with ABVD ($n = 24$) and found that 28/29 (97 percent) of MOPP chemotherapy patients were azoospermic after therapy. Remarkably, all patients treated with ABVD therapy were normozoospermic after a median of 10 months. Unsurprisingly, with a high cure rate, ABVD has now become the current gold standard treatment for Hodgkin's lymphoma and, although the low-risk approach is to refer all patients for sperm banking as a precaution, its continued use will no doubt reduce the need for sperm banking in this group of patients.

In a similar but slightly less dramatic way, the treatment for testicular cancer has been modified to reduce toxicity. Bleomycin, etoposide and cisplatin (BEP) remains standard therapy for nonseminomatous tumors and toxicity is attributed to the cumulative dose of cisplatin (Lampe *et al.*, 1997). Until recently, adjuvant therapy for low-grade seminomatous tumors was radiotherapy. However, azoospermia is a relatively common side effect and, of all treatments for testicular cancer, radiotherapy has the most negative impact on male fertility (Huyghe *et al.*, 2004). Lately, however, a single dose of carboplatin has been successfully employed, reducing relapse rates for either stages I and II seminoma, and showing very little gonadotoxicity (Reiter *et al.*, 1998; Patterson *et al.*, 2001; Steiner *et al.*, 2002). Of course, as with Hodgkin's lymphoma patients, the cautious approach is to refer the patient for sperm banking regardless of the relatively lower risk. As with all cancer therapies, priority must be given to relief of symptoms, prolonging life, and, in an increasing number of cases, a cure. However, as therapies become more successful attention becomes more focussed on making those therapies more tolerable and reducing their long-term side-effects. There has to be a sufficiently large body of evidence to demonstrate both a resumption of spermatogenesis and normal sperm DNA postchemotherapy to support whole-scale abandonment of sperm banking in this group, yet this remains a possibility in the future.

References

Aminsharifi, A.R., Talaei, T., Kumar, V. *et al.* (2007). A postulated role of testosterone for prevention of cisplatin gonadal toxicity. *Medical Hypotheses*, **68**, 525–7.

Anselmo, A.P., Cartoni, C., Bellantuono, P. *et al.* (1990). Risk of infertility in patients with Hodgkin's disease treated with ABVD vs. MOPP vs. ABVD/MOPP. *Haematologica*, **75**, 155–8.

Ben Arush, W.M., Solt, I., Lightman, A., Linn, S. & Kuten, A. (2000). Male gonadal function in survivors of childhood Hodgkin's and non-Hodgkin's lymphoma. *Pediatric Hematology and Oncology*, **17**, 239–45.

Boekelheide, K., Schoenfeld, H.A., Hall, S.J. *et al.* (2005). Gonadotropin-releasing hormone antagonist (cetrorelix) therapy fails to protect nonhuman primates (*Macaca arctoides*) from radiation-induced spermatogenic failure. *Journal of Andrology*, **26**, 222–34.

Bokemeyer, C., Berger, C.C., Kuczyk, M.A. & Schmoll, H.J. (1996). Evaluation of long-term toxicity after chemotherapy for testicular cancer. *Journal of Clinical Oncology*, **14**, 2923–32.

Bonadonna, G. (1982). Chemotherapy strategies to improve the control of Hodgkin's disease. *Cancer Research*, **42**, 4309–20.

Brinster, R.L. & Zimmermann, J.W., (1994). Spermatogenesis following male germ cell transplantation. *Proceedings of the National Academy of Sciences of the United States of America*, **91**, 11298–302.

Canellos, G.P., Anderson, J.R., Propert, K.L. et al. (1992). Chemotherapy of advanced Hodgkin's disease with MOPP, ABVD, or MOPP alternating with ABVD. *New England Journal of Medicine*, **327**, 1478–83.

Chapman, R.M., Sutcliffe, S.B., Rees, L.H. & Edwards, C.R.W. (1979). Cyclical combination chemotherapy and gonadal function: retrospective study in males. *Lancet*, **1**, 285–9.

Cozzi, E., Bosio, E., Seveso, M., Vadori, M. & Ancona, E. (2006). Xenotransplantation – current status and future perspectives. *British Medical Bulletin*, **75–76**, 99–114.

Department of Health (DoH). (2006). *Review of the Human Fertilisation and Embryology Act*. London: HMSO.

Dobrinski, I. (2005). Advances and applications of germ cell transplantation. *Human Fertility*, **9**, 9–14.

Drusenheimer, N., Wulf, G., Nolte, J. et al. (2007). Putative human male germ cells from bone marrow stem cells. *Society of Reproduction and Fertility Supplement*, **63**, 69–76.

Ellen, G. & Herman, T. (2007). Is there a clinical future for spermatogonial stem cells? *Current Stem Cell Research and Therapy*, **2**, 189–95.

Geijsen, N., Horoschak, M., Kim, K. et al. (2004). Derivation of embryonic germ cells and male gametes from embryonic stem cells. *Nature*, **427**, 148–54.

Georgiou, I., Pardalidis, N., Giannakis, D. et al. (2007). In vitro spermatogenesis as a method to bypass pre-meiotic or post-meiotic barriers blocking the spermatogenetic process: genetic and epigenetic implications in assisted reproductive technology. *Andrologia*, **39**, 159–76.

Hochi, S., Watanabe, K., Kato, M. & Hirabayashi, M. (2008). Live rats resulting from injection of oocytes with spermatozoa freeze-dried and stored for one year. *Molecular Reproduction and Development*, **75**, 890–4.

Honaramooz, A., Snedaker, A., Boiani, M. et al. (2002). Sperm from neonatal mammalian testes grafted in mice. *Nature*, **418**, 778–81.

Huleihel, M., Abuelhija, M. & Lunenfeld, E. (2007). In vitro culture of testicular germ cells: regulatory factors and limitations. *Growth Factors*, **25**, 236–52.

Huyghe, E., Matsuda, T., Daudin, M. et al. (2004). Fertility after testicular cancer treatments: results of a large multicenter study. *Cancer*, **15**, 732–7.

Jahnukainen, K., Hou, M., Petersen, C., Setchell, B. & Soder, O. (2001). Intratesticular transplantation of testicular cells from leukemic rats causes transmission of leukemia. *Cancer Research*. **61**, 706–10.

Johnson, D.S., Russell, L.D. & Griswold, M.D. (2000). Advances in spermatogonial stem cell transplantation. *Reviews of Reproduction*. **5**, 183–8.

Kantasu-Shinohara, M., Ogonuki, N., Inoue, K. et al. (2003). Restoration of fertility in infertile mice by transplantation of cryopreserved male germinal stem cells. *Human Reproduction*, **18**, 2660–7.

Kusakabe, H., Yanagimachi, R. & Kamiguchi, Y., (2007). Mouse and human spermatozoa can be freeze-dried without damaging their chromosomes. *Human Reproduction*, **23**, 233–9.

Lampe, H., Horwich, A., Norman, A., Nicholls, J. & Dearnaley, D.P. (1997). Fertility after chemotherapy for testicular germ cell cancers. *Journal of Clinical Oncology*, **15**, 239–45.

Liu, J.L., Kusakabe, H., Chang, C.C. et al. (2004). Freeze-dried sperm fertilization leads to full-term development in rabbits. *Biology of Reproduction*, **70**, 1776–81.

Masala, A., Faedda, R., Alagna, S. et al. (1997). Use of testosterone to prevent cyclophosphamide-induced azoospermia. *Annals of Internal Medicine*, **126**, 292–5.

Mitwally, M.F. (2007). Fertility preservation and minimizing reproductive damage in cancer survivors. *Expert Review of Anticancer Therapy*, 7, 989–1001.

Nagano, M., Patrizio, P. & Brinster, R.L. (2002). Long-term survival of human spermatogonial stem cells in mouse testes. *Fertility and Sterility*, **78**, 1225–33.

Nayernia, K., Nolte, J., Michelmann, H.W. et al. (2006). In vitro differentiated embryonic stem cells give rise to male gametes that can generate offspring in mice. *Developmental Cell*, **11**, 1–8.

Parks, J.E., Lee, D.R., Huang, S. & Kaproth, M. T. (2003). Prospects for spermatogenesis in vitro. *Theriogenology*, **59**, 73–86.

Patterson, H., Norman, A.R., Mitra, S.S. *et al.* (2001). Combination carboplatin and radiotherapy in the management of stage II testicular seminoma: comparison with radiotherapy treatment alone. *Radiotherapy and Oncology*, **59**, 5–11.

Radford, J., Shalet, S. & Lieberman, B. (1999). Fertility after treatment for cancer. Questions remain over ways of preserving ovarian and testicular tissue. *British Medical Journal*, **319**, 935–6.

Reiter, W.J., Kratzik, C., Brodowicz, T. *et al.* (1998). Sperm analysis and serum follicle-stimulating hormone levels before and after adjuvant single-agent carboplatin therapy for clinical stage I seminoma. *Urology* **52**, 117–19.

Schlatt, S. (2002). Germ cell transplantation. *Molecular and Cellular Endocrinology*, **186**, 163–7.

Schlatt, S., Honaramooz, A., Boiani, M., Schöler, H.R. & Dobrinski, I. (2003). Progeny from sperm obtained after ectopic grafting of neonatal mouse testes. *Biology of Reproduction*, **68**, 2331–5.

Shetty, G. & Meistrich, M.L. (2005). Hormonal approaches to preservation and restoration of male fertility after cancer treatment. *Journal of the National Cancer Institute. Monographs*, **34**, 36–9.

Steiner, H., Holtl, L., Wirtenberger, W. *et al.* (2002). Long-term experience with carboplatin monotherapy for clinical stage I seminoma: a retrospective single-center study. *Urology*, **60**, 324–8.

Tal, R., Botchan, A., Hauser, R. *et al.* (2000). Follow-up of sperm concentration and motility in patients with lymphoma. *Human Reproduction*, **15**, 1985–8.

Tesarik, J. & Mendoza, C. (2003). Somatic cell haploidization: an update. *Reproductive Biomedicine Online*, **6**, 60–5.

Toyooka, Y., Tsunekawa, N., Akasu, R. & Noce, T. (2003). Embryonic stem cells can form germ cells in vitro. *Proceedings of the National Academy of Sciences of the United States of America*, **100**, 11457–62.

Viviani, S., Santoro, A., Ragni, G. *et al.* (1985). Gonadal toxicity after combination chemotherapy for Hodgkin's disease. Comparative results of MOPP vs. ABVD. *European Journal of Cancer and Clinical Oncology*, **21**, 601–5.

Wakayama, T. & Yanagimachi, R. (1998). Development of normal mice from oocytes injected with freeze-dried spermatozoa. *Nature Biotechnology*, **16**, 639–641.

Wyns, C., Curaba, M., Martinez-Madrid, B. *et al.* (2007). Spermatogonial survival after cryopreservation and short-term orthotopic immature human cryptorchid testicular tissue grafting to immunodeficient mice. *Human Reproduction*, **22**, 1603–11.

Index

ABVD treatment for
  Hodgkin's lymphoma 23,
  24, 118–19
acrosome integrity, factors
  affecting 9
adolescent cancer patients
  sperm banking services
    41–2
  sperm retrieval methods 81
adolescents, legal and ethical
  issues 62–3
adriamycin 23, 24, 118–19
aggressive illness and sperm
  banking 41–2
alarm systems for sperm
  banks 102
alkylating agents
  ability to produce prolonged
    azoospermia 22, 23
  germ cell mutation
    induction 24
anejaculation (AE), sperm
  retrieval options 76
antineoplastic agents
  effects on reproductive
    function 18–19
  genetic mutations in germ
    cells 20, 24–5
  patient information about
    sperm banking 18
  recovery of spermatogenesis
    22–4
  see also chemotherapy;
    cytotoxic therapy;
    gonadotoxic therapy
artificial insemination (AI)
  and sperm cryopreservation
    1, 2–4
  history of development 1,
    2–4
assisted conception
  case reports 112
  choice of technique with
    banked sperm 108–10
  sperm selection methods
    111–12
  tests of sperm DNA quality
    111–12
  use of banked sperm 106

use of frozen or fresh
  (post-treatment) sperm
  110–11
assisted conception techniques
  107
  in vitro fertilisation (IVF)
    107–8
  intra cytoplasmic sperm
    injection (ICSI) 108,
    109
  intra-uterine insemination
    (IUI) 107
auditing of sperm bank
  inventory 100, 101
autoimmune disorders, patient
  information about sperm
  banking 18
autonomic dysreflexia (AD),
  risk with PVS for SCI
  patients 77
azoospermia
  effects of cancer treatment
    82
  effects of chemotherapy 21
  effects of particular
    chemotherapeutic
    agents 22–4
  effects of radiation doses
    22, 23
  prolonged effects of
    cytotoxic therapy
    22–4
  recovery after cytotoxic
    therapy 22–4

BEP therapy for testicular
  cancer 119
bleomycin 24, 118–19
Blood, Stephen, legal case over
  posthumous use of sperm
  64–8
boar sperm cryopreservation
  3, 9
bull sperm cryopreservation
  2, 9
  use of extenders 2

cancer, effects on reproductive
  function 18

cancer diagnosis
  patient information about
    sperm banking 18
  psychosocial impact
    42–4
  see also diagnosis of life-
    threatening illness
cancer patients
  coping with sperm banking
    43
  long-term impact of fertility
    issues 53–4
  research on reducing
    chemotherapy toxicity
    118–19
  sperm banking prior to
    therapy 73
  sperm banking services
    41–2
cancer treatment
  effects on reproductive
    function 18–19
  ejaculatory dysfunction
    caused by 82
  erectile dysfunction caused
    by 82
  indication for sperm
    cryopreservation
    10–11
  infertility risk 10–11
  natural fertility post-
    treatment 105, 106
  see also chemotherapy;
    cytotoxic therapy;
    radiotherapy
carboplatin 119
cattle, development of AI
  techniques 2 see also bull
  sperm cryopreservation
cell damage caused by
  cryopreservation 5–6
  see also DNA damage in
    sperm
chemotherapy
  effects on sperm count 22
  effects on sperm production
    21, 22
  research on reducing
    toxicity 118–19

sperm banking after
   initiation of 24–5
childhood cancer, fertility
   preservation research 81
children, legal and ethical
   issues 62–3
ChIVPP/PABlOE treatment
   for Hodgkin's lymphoma
   118–19
chlorambucil 118–19
chromatin damage in
   spermatozoa,
   measurement 25–6
chromosomal abnormalities in
   human sperm,
   measurement 25
cisplatin 22, 23, 105, 119
COMET assay 25–6, 111
communication about sperm
   banking
   at time of diagnosis 41
   decision making and consent
      45–6
   when and where to discuss it
      46–8
conception see assisted
   conception
consent to creation of embryos
   59, 60
consent to sperm banking
   impact of receiving
      diagnosis 45–6
   informed consent 41
   minors and adolescents
      62–3
   patient counseling on
      59–60
   range of public opinion on
      69–70
consent to sperm storage
   and future use 59–60,
   69–70
contact tracing by sperm banks
   38–9, 61
containment (packaging)
   systems for sperm
   cryopreservation 88–91
cooling rates for sperm, linear
   and non-linear 6–7
   see also fundamental
      cryobiology
coping strategies
   professional responses to
      50–1

responses to life-threatening
   illness 49–50
critically ill men, sperm
   cryopreservation 11–12
cryo-loop 7
cryobiology, history of 4
   see also fundamental
      cryobiology
cryopreservation protocols
   development of 4–7, 8
   experimental example 7–9
   research on species- or
      strain-specific protocols
      10
   see also sperm
      cryopreservation
cryoprotectant media 88
cryoprotective agents (CPAs)
   discovery of 4
   role in cryopreservation
      protocols 6
   vitrification protocols 7, 8
cyclophosphamide 18, 24
cytotoxic therapy
   effects of particular cytotoxic
      agents 22–4
   effects on offspring
      conceived after
      initiation 26
   effects on spermatozoa
      19, 20
   indication for sperm
      cryopreservation 10–11
   natural fertility post-
      treatment 105, 106
   permanent DNA damage in
      sperm 25–6
   recovery of spermatogenesis
      22–4
   see also chemotherapy;
      gonadotoxic therapy;
      radiotherapy

dacarbazine 24, 118–19
deceased men, sperm
   cryopreservation 11–12
decision making about sperm
   banking, impact of
   receiving diagnosis 45–6
diagnosis of life-threatening
   illness
   communication issues 41
   consent for sperm banking
      45–6

coping strategies 49–50
coping with 44–5
coping with sperm banking
   43
gender differences in
   reactions 43–4
impact on decision making
   45–6
obtaining informed
   consent 41
patient information about
   sperm banking 18
professional response to
   patients' coping
   strategies 50–1
psychosocial impact 42–4
responses to 49–50
differentiating spermatogonia
   19
effects of cytotoxic therapies
   19
dimethyl sulfoxide (DMSO),
   cryoprotective agent 6
DNA damage in sperm
   effects of cryopreservation
      110–11
   effects of cytotoxic therapy
      25–6
   effects of gonadotoxic
      therapy 110–11
   measurement 25–6
   quality testing 111–12
dogs, development of AI
   techniques 2
domestic species
   distribution of "genetically
      superior" lines 1
   preservation of genetic
      diversity 1
doxorubicin 118–19

early warning systems for
   sperm banks 102
egg yolk lipid extenders 2
ejaculatory dysfunction, effects
   of cancer treatment 82
electroejaculation (EEJ), sperm
   retrieval 77–8
embryos, consent to creation of
   59, 60
emotional context of sperm
   banking 51–3
endangered species, sperm
   cryopreservation 12

endocrine manipulation to protect the testis 115–16
erectile dysfunction (ED), effects of cancer treatment 82
ethical aspects of sperm banking
  adolescents 62–3
  consent 59–60, 69–70
  contact tracing 61
  length of period of storage 60–1
  minors 62–3
  posthumous use of stored sperm 58, 63–8, 69, 70
  rights to banked sperm 59–60
etoposide 24, 118–19
extender development for sperm cryopreservation 2

fertility, long-term impact of threats to 53–4
fertility preservation research
  alternatives to liquid nitrogen storage 118
  endocrine manipulation to protect the testis 115–16
  freeze-drying of sperm 118
  generation of artificial sperm 118
  gonadal tissue/cells freezing and re-transplantation 116
  reducing toxicity of chemotherapy 118–19
  sperm production in vitro 116–17
  xenotransplantation of reproductive tissues 117
FISH (fluorescence in situ hybridization) to measure chromosomal abnormalities 25
freeze-drying of sperm 9, 10, 118
freezing of sperm samples see sperm cryopreservation
fundamental cryobiology
  action of cryoprotective agents (CPAs) 6
  cryopreservation protocol development 4–7, 8

cryopreservation protocol experimental example 7–9
  definition and scope 4
  early work of Mazur 5–6
  effects of supercooling 5–6, 6–7
  history of cryobiology 4
  linear and non-linear cooling rates 6–7
  mechanisms of cell damage 5–6
  probability of intracellular ice formation (P_{IIF}) (Toner) 7, 8
  two-factor hypothesis (Mazur) 5–6
  vitrification 7, 8
funding issues for sperm banking 38
future developments see fertility preservation research

gender differences, coping with life-threatening illness 43–4
genetic diversity preservation 1
genetic mutation in germ cells
  effects of antineoplastic agents 20, 24–5
  susceptibility of stages of spermatogenesis 24
genetic mutation in human sperm 24–5, 20
  measurement 24–5
genetically engineered animal models (GEMs), sperm cryopreservation 1, 12
germ cells 19
  effects of cytotoxic therapies 19
  mutation induction by antineoplastic agents 20, 24–5
Gillick Competence 62–3
glycerol
  action in cryopreservation 6
  discovery of cryoprotective properties 1, 2, 4
  see also cryoprotective agents (CPAs)

gonadal tissue
  freezing and post-treatment re-transplantation 116
  research on xenotransplantation 117
gonadotoxic therapy, natural fertility post treatment 105, 106

handling of stored sperm samples 91, 92
history of sperm cryopreservation 1
  boar sperm 3
  bull sperm 2
  discovery of effects of glycerol 1, 2
  extender development 2
  human sperm 4
  link with development of AI 1, 2–4
  mouse sperm 3
Hodgkin's lymphoma (Hodgkin's disease)
  ABVD treatment 23, 24, 118–19
  research on reducing toxicity of chemotherapy 118–19
  toxicity of treatments 21, 23, 24
horses, development of AI techniques 2
Human Fertilisation and Embryology Act (1990) 58–9
Human Fertilisation and Embryology (Deceased Fathers) Bill (2003) 68
human sperm cryopreservation development 4
  cryopreservation research 10
  mutation induction by antineoplastic agents 20, 24–5
hydrocele 11

iatrogenic infertility risk, indication for sperm cryopreservation 1, 10–11
ICSI see intra cytoplasmic sperm injection

immunosuppressive therapy, indication for sperm cryopreservation 11
in situ nick translation test 111
in vitro fertilisation (IVF)
indications for sperm cryopreservation 11
technique 107–8
infertility treatment, indication for sperm cryopreservation 11
informed consent *see* consent to sperm banking
intra-uterine insemination (IUI)
indications for sperm cryopreservation 11
technique 107
intracellular ice formation model (Toner) 7, 8
intra cytoplasmic sperm injection (ICSI)
semen parameters for successful fertilization 73
semen quality 106
technique 108, 109
use with freeze-dried sperm 9, 10
IVF *see* in vitro fertilisation

labeling of stored sperm samples 92, 91
legal aspects of sperm banking
adolescents 62–3
case of Lance Smith 68
case of Stephen Blood 64–8
consent 59–60, 69–70
contact tracing 61
distinction between rights and desires 70
Gillick Competence 62–3
Human Fertilisation and Embryology Act (1990) 58–9
legal frameworks 58–9
length of period of storage 60–1
minors 62–3
posthumous use of stored sperm 58, 63–8, 69, 70
rights to banked sperm 59–60

UK legal framework 58–9
welfare of the potential child 69
leukemia in childhood, fertility preservation research 81
Leydig cells 18–19
life-threatening illness *see* diagnosis of life-threatening illness
liquid nitrogen storage of sperm *see* sperm storage (long-term)
long-term impacts of threat to fertility 53–4
L_p (water permeability of a cell membrane) 8, 10

masturbatory ejaculates, sperm retrieval 73–6
mechlorethamine 118–19
medical barriers to sperm banking 41–2
medical disciplines, interface with the sperm bank 30
microsurgical epididymal sperm aspiration (MESA) 81
minisatellite mutations in human sperm 24–5
minors, legal and ethical issues 62–3
monitoring systems for sperm banks 102
MOPP treatment for Hodgkin's lymphoma 23, 24
MOPP/ABV treatment for Hodgkin's lymphoma 118–19
moral issues related to sperm banking 41
motivations for sperm banking 48–9
mouse sperm cryopreservation research 10
results in inbred strains 3
variable success among genotypes 3

natural fertility after gonadotoxic therapy 105, 106
nephrotic disorders, patient information about sperm banking 18

nitrogen mustard 23, 24

osmotic tolerance limits (OTLs) of sperm 10
osmotically inactive portion of a cell (V_b) 8

partial zona dissection (PZD) technique 108
patient counseling on the implications of consent 59–60
patient information about sperm banking 18
easing stress and uncertainty 51–3
for sperm banking referral 34–8
when and where to discuss 46–8
patient referral for sperm banking
arrangements for long-term contact 38–9
barriers to referral 30–1
barriers to successful banking 30
funding issues 38
guidelines for referral 33, 34, 35
identifying men at risk of infertility 32–3
patient information 34–8
patients who cannot attend the sperm bank 38
problem areas 38–9
sources of medical referrals 30–1
timescale 32–3
unconscious patients 38
very ill patients 38
penile vibratory stimulation (PVS), sperm retrieval 75, 77, 78
percutaneous epididymal sperm aspiration (PESA) 79
poor prognosis and sperm banking 41–2
posthumous use of stored sperm
case of Lance Smith 68
case of Stephen Blood 64–8

posthumous use of stored
    sperm (*cont.*)
  conception by a surrogate
    68
  differences in national laws
    63–4
  factors to consider 64
  legal and ethical aspects 58,
    63–8, 69, 70
  range of public opinion on
    70
  views among different
    religions 63–4
  welfare of the potential child
    69
post-mortem sperm retrieval
    (PMSR) 11–12
prednisolone 118–19
prednisone 24
probability of intracellular ice
    formation (P_{IIF}) (Toner)
    7, 8
procarbazine 24, 23, 118–19
professionals
  response to patient coping
    strategies 50–1
  skills development and
    maintenance 41
P_s (solute permeability of a cell
    membrane) 8, 10
psychological impact of sperm
    banking 41–2
psychosocial impact of cancer
    diagnosis 42–4
public opinion
  on consent 69–70
  on posthumous use of sperm
    70

radiotherapy
  decision to bank sperm 22
  effects on sperm production
    21–2
  permanent DNA damage in
    sperm 25–6
  see also cytotoxic therapy;
    gonadotoxic therapy
radiation, induction of germ-
    cell mutation 24
referral *see* patient referral for
    sperm banking
religious views on posthumous
    use of stored sperm
    63–4

retrograde ejaculation (RE)
  causes 76
  effects of cancer treatment 82
  sperm retrieval 76–7

sample safety in sperm banks
    101–2
semen analysis 86–7
semen quality
  post treatment 105, 106
  use of ICSI 106
seminiferous (germinal)
    epithelium 19
Sertoli cells 19
service evaluation in sperm
    banking services 39
single cell electrophoresis test 111
Smith, Lance, legal case over
    posthumous use of sperm
    68
solute permeability of a cell
    membrane (P_s) 8, 10
species- or strain-specific
    cryopreservation
    protocols 10
sperm
  effects of cytotoxic therapies
    19, 20
  persistent DNA damage in
    25–6
  see also human sperm
sperm bank, interface with
    medical disciplines 30
sperm banking
  after initiation of
    chemotherapy 24–5
  barriers to provision 41–2
  challenges of service
    provision 41–2
  decision prior to
    radiotherapy 22
  experience of service users
    51–3
  importance of early
    information about 18
  long-term impact of
    decisions about 53–4
  motivations for decision to
    use 48–9
  recommendation for cancer
    patients 73
  service evaluation 39
  services for younger cancer
    patients 41–2

when and where to discuss
    with patients 46–8
sperm chromatin structure
    assay (SCSA) 25–6
sperm count
  effects of chemotherapy 22
  effects of radiation doses
    22, 23
sperm cryopreservation
  containment (packaging)
    systems 88–91
  cryoprotectant media 88
  egg yolk lipid extenders 2
  freezing 92–3, 94
  genetically modified animal
    models 1
  handling 91, 92
  importance in iatrogenic
    infertility 1
  labeling 91, 92
  range of functions 1
  semen analysis 86–7
  sperm processing prior to
    freezing 87–8
  stages in the process 86, 87
  variable success among
    mammalian species 1
  see also cryopreservation
    protocols; sperm
    storage
sperm cryopreservation
    indications
  cancer treatment infertility
    risk 10–11
  critically ill or deceased men
    11–12
  cytotoxic therapies 10–11
  endangered species 12
  genetically engineered
    animal models (GEMs)
    12
  iatrogenic infertility risk
    10–11
  immunosuppressive
    therapies 11
  infertility treatment 11
  surgery for reproductive
    problems 11
sperm cryopreservation
    research 9–10
  boar sperm
    cryopreservation 9
  bull sperm
    cryopreservation 9

factors affecting acrosome integrity 9
freeze-drying of sperm 9, 10
human sperm cryopreservation 10
loss of sperm motility 9, 10
mouse sperm cryopreservation 10
osmotic tolerance limits (OTLs) of sperm 10
species- or strain-specific protocols 10
sperm DNA see DNA damage in sperm
sperm motility loss 9, 10
sperm processing prior to freezing 87–8
sperm retrieval, semen quality for successful fertilisation 73, 76
sperm retrieval methods
adolescents 81
after medical treatment 81–2
electroejaculation (EEJ) 77–8
masturbatory ejaculates 73–6
microsurgical epididymal sperm aspiration (MESA) 81
options with anejaculation (AE) 76
penile vibratory stimulation (PVS) 75, 77, 78
percutaneous epididymal sperm aspiration (PESA) 79
post treatment azoospermia 82
post treatment ejaculatory dysfunction 82
post treatment erectile dysfunction 82
range of options 73, 74
retrograde ejaculation (RE) 76–7
risk of autonomic dysreflexia (AD) 77
seminal collection device (non-spermicidal condom) 74–5
surgical sperm retrieval (SSR) 78–81

testicular sperm aspiration (TESA) 79–80
testicular sperm extraction (TESE) 79–80
sperm selection for assisted conception 111–12
sperm storage
containment (packaging) systems 88–91
design of freezer furniture (racking) 94–5
handling 92, 91
labeling 91, 92
sperm storage (long-term)
alarm systems 102
alternatives to liquid nitrogen 118
auditing of inventory 100, 101
early warning systems 102
liquid nitrogen or vapour phase 95–7
maintaining nitrogen supply 98–9, 100
monitoring systems 102
research on freeze-drying of sperm 118
sample safety 101–2
staff safety 100–1
storage period for sperm 60–1
spermatids 19
spermatocytes 19
spermatogenesis
arrangement of cells in the testis 19
cells involved in 19
effects of chemotherapy 21, 22
effects of cytotoxic therapies 19, 20
effects of radiotherapy 21–2
kinetics of differentiation 20
normal process 19–20
recovery after cytotoxic therapy 22–4
research on generation of artificial sperm 118
research on in vitro sperm production 116–17
susceptibility to mutation induction 24

spinal cord injury (SCI) patients, PVS sperm retrieval method 75, 77, 78
staff safety at sperm banks 100–1
stem spermatogonia 19
cell transplantation research 116, 117
subzonal insemination (SUZI) technique 108
supercooling, effects on cells 5–6, 6–7
surgical sperm retrieval (SSR) 78–81
surrogate, conception by 68

teenage cancer patients see adolescent cancer patients
testicular cancer
BEP therapy 119
research on reducing toxicity of chemotherapy 119
testicular sperm aspiration (TESA) 79–80
testicular sperm extraction (TESE) 79–80
testis
arrangement of cells 19
effects of cytotoxic therapies 19
effects of radiation dose on sperm count 22, 23
endocrine manipulation to protect 115–16
radiation dose from various treatments 21–2
testosterone levels, effects of cytotoxic therapies 18–19
transurethral resection of the ejaculatory ducts (TURED) 11
Tris–egg yolk–glycerol method for freezing sperm 2
TUNEL assay 25–6, 111
two-factor hypothesis (Mazur) 5–6

varicocele 11
V_b (osmotically inactive portion of a cell) 8
vinblastine 23, 24, 118–19

vincristine 24, 118–19
vitrification 7, 8

Warnock Committee 58–9
water permeability of a cell
    membrane (L_p) 8, 10

wild species, preservation of
    genetic diversity 1

xenotransplantation of
    reproductive tissues
    117

younger patients *see* adolescent
    cancer patients; children;
    minors

zona drilling (ZD) technique
    108